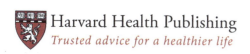

Dear Reader,

Many people are concerned about their hearing, and rightly so. Hearing connects us to other people, and the loss of hearing can lead to isolation and withdrawal from many pleasurable activities. Hearing ability declines with age. The National Institute on Deafness and Other Communication Disorders estimates that age-related hearing loss affects nearly 25% of adults ages 65 to 74 and 50% of people 75 or older.

Hearing loss has many causes, including genetic defects, infection, and side effects from medication, but one cause is avoidable: about a third of cases are the result of routine exposure to very loud noise. Most baby boomers have been exposed to plenty of loud music, not to mention the noise of leaf blowers, sirens, blow dryers, and other loud equipment. Still, studies show that people now in their 60s have better hearing than their parents did at that age, probably as a result of better noise protection in the workplace in industries such as manufacturing.

The good news for anyone struggling to hear is that hearing aids and surgical options have improved tremendously. If you weren't a good candidate for a hearing aid five years ago, come back and try again. Digital hearing aids are better, more powerful, and small enough to be barely noticeable, and their technology continually improves. They do a better job of managing sounds—that is, boosting the sounds you want to hear and reducing the impact of the ones you don't, such as the background noise in a restaurant.

What's more, new wireless technologies are also improving, enabling you to hear better than you ever could before in various situations—on the phone, watching TV, or even in a public venue, such as a movie theater, auditorium, or train station. New apps enable you to wirelessly control the settings of your hearing aids with your phone and to stream music and phone calls directly into your hearing aids. If you are not a candidate for a traditional hearing aid, other technologies such as an implantable device or surgery may be helpful.

Beginning in 2020, new over-the-counter hearing aids will also be available, although they won't have the sophistication of the customized hearing aids discussed in this report. Think of them as the audiological equivalent of the generic reading glasses available at your pharmacy.

Of course, it's best to stop hearing loss from occurring in the first place. But even if you already have some hearing loss, it's not too late to prevent further damage. Wear earplugs when using noisy equipment. Moderate the volume on your music player. And pass along this information to your children and grandchildren to help keep their world sounding crisp and clear.

Sincerely,

David Murray Vernick, M.D.
Medical Editor

Ann Gentili-Stockwell, M.A., CCC-A
Medical Editor

Harvard Health Publishing | Harvard Medical School | 4 Blackfan Circle, 4th Floor | Boston, MA 02115

How we hear

Because hearing seems automatic, we take it for granted until it is impaired. But the process of hearing is truly awe-inspiring. The ear is a precision instrument with an astonishingly intricate mechanism, and the journey of sound through the ear is the stuff of adventure, involving navigation through air and water, and even, metaphorically speaking, moving boulders.

The journey of sound

The tale begins when a person speaks, a musician strikes a chord, or some other noise occurs. The sound, in the form of sound waves, travels through the air, then follows the swirling channel of the outer ear into the ear canal. The ear canal is a dark, slippery passageway, a mere inch long. It's slippery because it's lined with earwax, a material secreted by glands in the ear canal that helps protect the ear by keeping out unwanted substances like bacteria and dirt.

The ear canal acts like an amplifier, boosting the sound's volume as it funnels sound to the eardrum—a slender skinlike structure about a half-inch across and the width of a strand of hair. Although small, the eardrum, also known as the tympanic membrane, forms a tight barrier that separates the outer ear from the middle ear (see Figure 1, below).

Sounding the drum

Like a drummer beating a drum, sound waves strike the eardrum and make it vibrate. The purpose of the eardrum is to boost the volume of incoming sound so that you can hear it comfortably (see Figure 2, page 3).

While the amplitude of a sound wave determines the loudness of a sound, the frequency of the vibrations determines the pitch. For example, a sound wave that vibrates at 256 cycles per second, like the middle C on the piano, is said to have a frequency of 256 hertz (Hz), the unit in which frequencies are measured. The higher the frequency of the sound wave, the higher the pitch will be (see "What is sound?" on page 4).

Figure 1: The outer, middle, and inner ear

The outer ear consists of the parts you can see: the fleshy outer part (called the auricle), the ear canal, and the eardrum.

The middle ear is an air-filled cavity containing the ossicles, three small bones (malleus, incus, and stapes) that transmit vibrations to the inner ear.

The inner ear is a complex system of membranous canals protected by a bony casing. Inside, the spiral-shaped cochlea contains the hair cells that transmit sound to the auditory nerve, which conducts sound to the brain. The vestibular system, which regulates balance, is also part of the inner ear and includes the three semicircular canals, which form the largest part of the labyrinth.

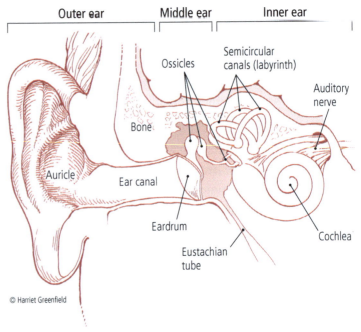

© Harriet Greenfield

As the eardrum vibrates, it transfers sound waves to the middle ear, which is an air-filled chamber about the size of a peanut. There, the sound waves encounter the ossicles, three bones that form a bridge across the middle ear. These three bones have Latin names that describe their shapes: the malleus (hammer), incus (anvil), and stapes (stirrup). The tiny sound waves must move these bony structures, causing them to vibrate—the part of the adventure akin to moving boulders.

Natural volume control

In the middle ear, the volume of the sound can be either increased or decreased. In most cases, the ossicles vibrate rapidly to boost the volume. They are aligned in such a way that this happens automatically. If the noise is too loud, however, two middle-ear muscles attached to the ossicles work to lower the volume: as these muscles contract, they pull on the three bones, reducing their ability to vibrate and preventing extremely loud noises from hurting your ears.

The vibrating ossicles transfer the sound-wave vibrations to the "oval window" that separates the middle ear from the inner ear. This window consists of the stapes footplate and a fibrous membrane that holds the footplate in place and seals the chamber.

The inner chamber

The inner ear houses the cochlea, a snail-shaped structure consisting of bone on the outside and fluid-filled membranes on the inside. As sound waves undulate through the liquid passageways, they send a ripple across rows of sensory cells, called hair cells, lining the cochlea. There are 10,000 to 15,000 hair cells in each ear, and sound waves of different frequencies stimulate the hair cells in different sections of the cochlea. Hair cells at the base (entrance) of the cochlea are stimulated by the higher frequencies, and those at the apex (center) of the cochlea are stimulated by lower frequencies. As the hairlike prongs on the hair cells bend, a chemical signal prompts the auditory nerve to relay a message to the brain, noting a particular sound's frequency and volume. The message goes to a section of the brain called the auditory cortex.

Although sound waves must pass through the different structures of the ear, the entire process—from

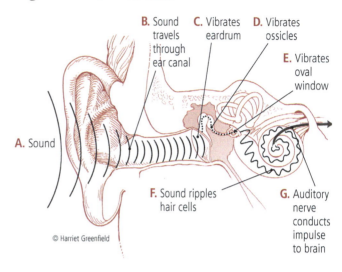

Figure 2: How we hear

Sound travels in waves through the air (**A**) into the ear canal (**B**), where it is amplified and causes the eardrum to vibrate (**C**). The eardrum transfers the vibrations to the tiny bones known as ossicles (**D**), which in turn transmit the vibrations through the membrane-covered opening called the oval window (**E**) and into the fluid in the cochlea in the inner ear. The cochlear fluid moves in waves, setting in motion the sensory hair cells inside the organ (**F**). The hair cells release electrochemical signals that travel along more than 30,000 auditory nerve pathways into the brain (**G**).

the moment a sound is made to the moment it reaches the brain—is practically instantaneous.

What you hear (and don't hear)

The arrival of auditory signals in the brain may seem like the end of the journey, but your brain still has to process the signals. Here the remarkable capabilities of the human brain are on display, for the brain does more than tell you what sound you just heard—which musical note was played, which word was spoken, and so on. It also sorts out the incoming sounds by their relative importance. The purpose is to tune out unimportant sounds, such as the flush of a toilet, the hum of the refrigerator, or the din in a restaurant, so that the sounds you really want to hear, like human voices, come through clearly. It's not that you don't hear the unimportant sounds; rather, your brain makes sure you don't notice them as much as the more significant sounds.

With age, however, your brain becomes less skilled at helping you ignore unwanted background noises.

What is sound?

Sound is a vibration of molecules that moves in the form of waves. Sound waves travel quickly, at about 770 mph in air. There are two measurable qualities that influence how we perceive sound. One is pitch (how high or low it is). The other is intensity (how loud it is).

A sound's pitch is determined by its frequency, or the number of cycles a sound wave makes in one second. The number of cycles is measured in hertz (abbreviated Hz). The higher the frequency of a sound, the higher the pitch. High-pitched sounds, such as a the high notes on a piano, have frequencies of thousands of hertz. Low-pitched sounds, such as thunder, have frequencies of only a few dozen hertz. People with normal hearing can hear frequencies as low as 20 and as high as 20,000 Hz. However, humans are most sensitive to sounds in the frequency range characteristic of human speech, 500 to 8,000 Hz.

A sound's intensity is determined by its amplitude, or the height of its sound wave. It is measured in decibels (dB). Decibels are not uniform units of measurement, like feet or yards, but rather a logarithmic progression. Therefore, an increase of 10 dB does not indicate the addition of 10 units, but rather a multiplication to 10 times the original level. The softest sound that an adult with normal hearing can hear is 0 dB, and the loudest sound, the deafening roar of a rocket taking off nearby, is more than 180 dB.

A third quality of sound, which is not measured by any specific unit, is timbre, or tone. It is timbre that helps you distinguish between different types of sounds, such as voices and musical instruments, even when they have the same frequency and intensity. For example, musical instruments produce more than just the "dominant frequency" that determines the pitch you hear; they also produce overtones, or secondary sound waves at different frequencies that give each instrument its distinct tone. In addition, instruments vary in the attack, sustain, and decay of the sound waves they produce.

This is not hearing loss per se, but a cognitive decline. Your brain simply doesn't process as efficiently as it once did, so its ability to diminish unwanted sound lessens. Here's one way to understand the difference between the brain of a teenager and that of a 60-year-old: the teenager can do his homework while the TV is on and his sister is talking loudly on the phone in the next room. An older person might have trouble concentrating on a television show if another person in the room is talking at even a normal volume.

A balancing act

Hearing isn't the ear's only job. The inner ear also contains the body's balance mechanism, which is why problems with balance and hearing often go hand in hand.

The balance mechanism, called the vestibular system, is housed in a structure called the labyrinth. The labyrinth consists of a maze of bone and tissue, with the cochlea (the hearing organ) at one end. At the other end are three fluid-filled loops called the semicircular canals, which are set at different angles (see Figure 1, page 2). At the base of each loop, a bell-shaped structure called a cupula sits above a clump of sensory hair cells like those in the cochlea. As fluid (endolymph) in a semicircular canal moves, its cupula tilts, bending the hair cells. Signals set off by this action travel to the brain via the acoustic nerve, telling it the position and rotational movements of your head—straight up and down (nodding "yes"), side to side (shaking your head "no"), tilting toward one shoulder, and so forth.

Between the cochlea and the semicircular canals are two additional sensory organs called the utricle and the saccule. These pouches are also lined with sensory hair cells that inform the brain about head position. Grains of calcium carbonate (called canaliths or otoconia) rest on top of a layer of gel overlying the hair cells. Each time your head tilts, gravity pulls on these tiny stones. Hair cells shift in response, sending signals to the brain that describe the position of your head. The sensory cells in the utricle also report forward motion—say, when you're walking or riding a bike. Those in the saccule monitor vertical acceleration, which would occur if you stood up or rode in an elevator, for example.

These five sensory organs in each inner ear provide the brain with enough information on the position and motion of your head that you can maintain your balance the vast majority of the time. However, if you spin around very fast, the fluid in the utricle and saccule can't move fast enough to tell your brain your exact position, so you feel dizzy.

When hearing loss occurs

You're having a meeting in a quiet room with a few people, and you can hear just about everything they say. Later, you're in a noisy restaurant and someone at your table tells a joke—you know it's a joke because everyone is laughing. You laugh, too, even though you haven't heard enough to understand the joke. This experience is typical of people whose hearing has begun to decline, especially those whose hearing loss is age-related, noise-related, or a combination of the two.

Hearing loss usually comes on so gradually, over so many years, that it can be hard to realize that you don't hear as well as you used to. The difference at first may not be so noticeable because people have a marvelous capacity to compensate for what they can't hear. For example, you may fill in gaps by picking up on the facial expressions and gestures of the person talking.

Although the term "hearing loss" implies trouble hearing all sounds, this may not be the case for you, especially early on. In fact, most people start off having trouble hearing just certain sounds. People with age-related hearing loss usually have most trouble hearing high-frequency, low-decibel sounds like a hiss, a whisper, or the "s" or "th" sounds that begin a word. In practical terms, what this means is that you can hear the vowels just fine, but consonants like "f" and "th" give you trouble. You might not be able to tell whether someone said "fish" or "this," "thing" or "sing." And you may have trouble hearing over the phone or when there's a lot of background noise. In a quiet room, you may do just fine.

As years pass, high-frequency sounds become harder to hear, even when the room is quiet. The doorbell or the telephone may ring and ring before you notice it. Lower-frequency sounds can also become problematic over time. You may find yourself increasingly asking others to repeat themselves, or holding back from conversation to avoid embarrassment.

Types of hearing loss

There are two basic types of hearing loss—sensorineural and conductive. Many people have a combination, especially as they age. These people are said to have mixed hearing loss. Knowing which type of hearing loss you have is the first step in determining which treatment is right for you.

Sensorineural hearing loss. More than 80% of people who are hard of hearing have sensorineural hearing loss. This type of hearing loss is caused by damage to the sensory cells (hair cells) in the ear or to the nerves that help transmit sound messages to the brain. Sensory cells can be injured or killed off by loud noises, toxic drugs, head injuries, and, above all, aging. When sensorineural hearing loss is the result of aging or an ongoing exposure to loud noise, it comes on gradually, over a period of many years. But it can start suddenly when the cause is a head injury, a toxic drug, or an extremely loud noise, such as an explosion. Sensorineural hearing loss is usually permanent.

Conductive hearing loss. This type of hearing loss is caused by something that physically blocks or hinders sound waves from passing through the outer ear or the middle ear. The source of the obstruction can be any number of things:

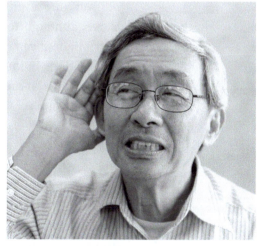

The term "hearing loss" implies trouble hearing all sounds, but most people with age-related hearing loss have trouble with high-frequency, low-decibel sounds, like a hiss, a whisper, or sounds like "th."

earwax, an accumulation of fluid, inflammation from an ear infection, a cyst or other abnormal growth, or a foreign body that becomes lodged accidentally in the ear. Conductive hearing loss can also be caused by disorders of the ossicles, such as otosclerosis. The eardrum itself can bring on conductive hearing loss if it becomes stretched or bruised from unequal air pressure in the middle ear, as might happen during changes in atmospheric pressure in an airplane. Sometimes the blockage is caused by a birth defect in which the ears don't develop properly.

Unlike sensorineural hearing loss, conductive hearing loss is often treatable with medicine or surgery. For example, you can remove excess earwax with a cleaning kit used at home, or you can ask your doctor to remove it.

Causes of hearing loss

Why do some people become hard of hearing while others live their entire lives without having to strain to hear? Various problems can harm the ear and impair hearing. For some people, there is a single, straightforward cause of hearing loss, like an accident or a severe infection. For others, the cause is not an experience but a genetic predisposition; the tendency to become hard of hearing with age runs in families. Many genetic mutations are known to cause hearing loss. But more often than not, it's a combination of experiences and genetics. Following are some of the main causes of hearing loss.

Presbycusis

Presbycusis, or age-related hearing loss, is the leading cause of hearing impairment. Over time, some hair cells in the inner ear grow old and die, and they are not replaced. When hair cells die, the electrical messages of sound waves don't travel to the brain as well as they should. The first hair cells to deteriorate are usually those that receive high-frequency sounds (see Figure 3, at left).

Everyone eventually gets presbycusis to some degree, although for many people its impact is relatively minor. It can mean that you have trouble hearing conversations in loud settings, for example. However, in severe cases, it can be difficult even to hear conversations in quiet places, and you might need a hearing aid.

Loud noises

Exposure to loud noises can cause sensorineural hearing loss in multiple ways. It can damage the hair cells in the inner ear. Alternatively, it can make the nerves in the cochlea swell, or it can increase the risk of an acoustic neuroma, a benign tumor on the nerve that connects the ears to the brain (see "Acoustic neuroma," page 11). Loud noise also increases the risk of

Continued on page 8

Figure 3: Age-related changes in hearing

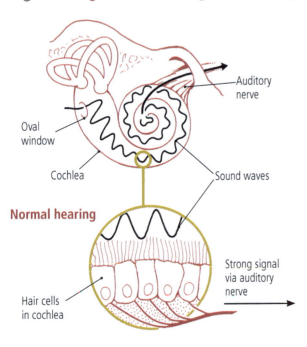

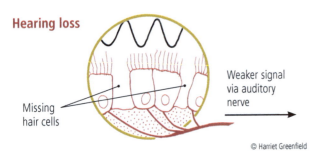

Age-related hearing loss usually results from damage to the tiny hair cells of the cochlea. Age and cumulative exposure to loud noise gradually damage these hair cells, and eventually the cells die. This leaves fewer cells to respond to sounds and thus causes hearing loss.

Tinnitus: Ringing in the ear

Many people with hearing loss also have tinnitus, commonly known as ringing in the ear. This phrase is misleading, however, because some people hear ringing while others hear whistles, chirping, or a combination of sounds. Regardless of the particular sound, the distinguishing feature is that it doesn't have an external cause. People with tinnitus hear sounds that people around them don't hear. This isn't to say that tinnitus isn't real—researchers at the National Institute on Deafness and Other Communication Disorders have detected changes in brain activity that occur with tinnitus.

Nearly everyone has had tinnitus for a few seconds or minutes after hearing a very loud noise. For example, using a snowmobile or lawn mower or attending a loud concert might trigger ringing in the ears. But one in five people has tinnitus on more than just a temporary basis. It's especially common in people over age 55, affecting about one in three people in this age group. It can occur in one or both ears.

The course of tinnitus is unpredictable. In some people, the symptoms remain the same over time; in others, they worsen. Just how severe tinnitus is seems to depend on a person's overall physical and mental health. In other words, the worse a person's health is, the worse the tinnitus is likely to be. As many as half of those with tinnitus also suffer from depression. In some cases, tinnitus contributes to depression, but in others, it may be a symptom.

Tinnitus tends to be worse in a quiet room, where there are few outside noises to mask the noise inside a person's head. This is why tinnitus sometimes causes insomnia. Most people develop strategies for coping with tinnitus, but for about 1% of people with the condition, it becomes so disabling that they have trouble functioning every day. These people need medical help and psychological counseling to handle the effects of the condition.

Causes of tinnitus

For most people with tinnitus, the cause is unknown. But many of the same things that cause hearing loss also cause tinnitus: loud noise, medications that are toxic to the nerves in the ear (see "Medications," page 10), impacted earwax, middle ear problems (such as infections and vascular tumors), and aging. Tinnitus is also a symptom of Ménière's disease (a disorder of the balance mechanism in the inner ear) and perilymph fistula (a hole in the inner ear). Many people say that it comes on when they are under stress.

When tinnitus has a physical cause, it can often be relieved with surgery or other treatments, like antibiotics to fight an ear infection or removal of impacted earwax. But the main treatment is counseling to assure people that tinnitus is not dangerous and to help them deal with the symptoms. There are also coping strategies that can reduce stress and help individuals learn to relax.

Strategies that can help

Some people with hearing loss and tinnitus find that both problems improve after they get a hearing aid or have a cochlear implant. Others find that their tinnitus symptoms improve somewhat when they cut down on caffeine and alcohol, reduce the amount of fat in their diets, and quit smoking. The following techniques may also help reduce your tinnitus symptoms:

- When you're in a quiet room, put on music or use a "white noise" machine. Background noise tends to drown out tinnitus sounds.

- Use the "tinnitus masker" on your hearing aid. This is a separate feature that is embedded into most hearing aids that allows you to choose a sound to "mask" the tinnitus sound you are hearing. How effective they are varies from person to person, but they usually do provide some level of relief for most people. Depending on the hearing aid, sounds that you could choose from may include spa music, chimes, white noise, and more. You can choose the pitch and loudness of the sound to suit your needs, and you can choose to turn it on or off.

- Tinnitus retraining therapy is an effective method for treating tinnitus, especially in people with tinnitus and oversensitive hearing. It is a lengthy, expensive process, taking 18 to 24 months, that relies on the principle of habituation, which occurs when your brain is exposed to a background sound, such as white noise, for long periods of time. After a while, the brain starts to filter out that particular background noise. Retraining therapy involves listening to a tone that is similar to the tinnitus sound for hours at a time. Eventually, your brain ignores the tone, along with the tinnitus sound.

- Reduce stress by whatever methods work for you. Try mindfulness meditation, which helps you learn not to focus on irritations such as the sound of tinnitus. Also try yoga, visualization, or other relaxation techniques.

- Consider biofeedback or hypnosis. Ask your doctor to recommend qualified practitioners.

Many of the same things that cause hearing loss also cause tinnitus, including loud noises and medications that are toxic to the ear nerves.

Continued from page 6

tinnitus, or ringing in the ears. How much damage is done depends on the loudness of the noise and how long it lasts, as well as a person's sensitivity to the ill effects of loud sounds. Spending a night at a loud rock concert can cause temporary hearing loss that lasts for several hours or several days. But going to loud concerts on a regular basis can cause cumulative damage to hair cells that leads to permanent hearing loss. And the increasing use of headphones and earbuds to listen to music may not bode well for lovers of loud music.

That said, several NIH-funded studies tracking hearing loss have found that the original rock-and-roll generation—baby boomers—have better hearing than their parents had at their age. The explanation is likely a combination of advances in public health, such as better sanitation (resulting in fewer ear infections) and better protection against noise in the workplace. Researchers noted decreasing occupational noise exposure from 1979 to 1999 in U.S. manufacturing and service industries, directly resulting from federally mandated changes designed to protect workers from the dangers of loud noise. The researchers also cited the decline of employment in manufacturing.

Exposure to one extremely loud noise, such as a bomb explosion, can cause permanent hearing loss.

CHUCK'S STORY: Staying connected

The onset of hearing loss as a young adult had a dramatic impact on the life of Chuck Scott, now 74. Back then, he was weeks away from graduating from college and was being drafted to serve in Vietnam. During his physical for Uncle Sam, however, he learned that his hearing was "bad enough that the military didn't want me," he says. For him that was a relief. He could pursue what would become a lifelong passion—a career in film editing.

Chuck didn't seek help for his hearing until the late 1970s, when his hearing had deteriorated to the point that it made his job difficult. "I was hearing the sound of voices, but not what people said," he explains. "I had to ask people over and over again to repeat themselves. It became a real problem."

Chuck received his first hearing aid when he was 30 years old—a large behind-the-ear model. If he was put off by the size, that disappointment was well offset by his restored ability to do his job well. "I'd wear my hearing aids all the time, even when I slept," he says. "I always wanted to be a part of everything that was going on, because when you are not hearing, you are isolated."

Two decades later, however, he'd lost virtually all of his natural hearing in his right ear, and what remained in his left ear had seriously degraded. It was around this time that he was diagnosed with otosclerosis, the leading cause of conductive hearing loss in young and middle-aged adults. Fortunately, hearing in his left ear was saved with a successful stapedectomy (see page 41). Surgery on his right ear did not help, but hearing aids did.

When digital hearing aids became available, Chuck was quick to buy one for his right ear that could filter out background noise. "It was a quantum leap forward," he says. "If I had meetings, I found that I could sit anywhere in the room rather than right next to the person who was speaking." With each advance in digital hearing aids, he has been able to hear better and in a broader range of situations. His most recent hearing aid, purchased nearly two years ago, allowed him to experience something he never thought would be possible—musical sound without distortion. "I have no hearing at frequencies higher than 3,000 Hz," he explains. "My new hearing aid shifts higher-frequency sounds to a lower frequency that is within my range of hearing. I don't know how it does that, but it has made a tremendous difference in the way I hear music and the understandability of certain sounds in speech that I have always struggled with."

Unfortunately, the trade-off is that the new hearing aid does not suppress background noise in restaurants as well. As a result, he sometimes will switch to an older hearing aid when he goes out to eat. Still, he is enthusiastic about the possibilities that hearing aids have opened up to him over the years, and he looks forward to the day when the latest hearing aids will combine all these features and strengths, so that he can meet his goal of hearing as naturally as possible.

For those who are not sure their hearing loss warrants a hearing aid and are reluctant to get tested, he has this to say: "A lot of people think that hearing aids are only for old people, and that's unfortunate because it's really not the case. I see people of all ages with hearing aids. What's worse is not being part of the conversation. You begin to become isolated, without even realizing it, and your quality of life starts to diminish." If that's not motivation enough, he says, consider your friends and family. If you can't hear them properly, "you will wind up checking out and shutting them out," as he puts it. "You will be missing out, but so will they."

Studies have implicated air bags. Some people whose lives were saved by air bags during car crashes have become partially or totally deaf as a result of the 170-dB sound made when an air bag is deployed. Cars sold in the United States are more likely to cause the problem because they are required to have larger, more powerful air bags than cars sold elsewhere.

More often than not, however, the noise that causes sensorineural hearing loss is not one deafening bang but decades' worth of exposure to the high-decibel accessories of daily life: leaf blowers, car horns, highway traffic, movie theater sounds, hair dryers, vacuum cleaners, loud music, and so on. Hair cells can break and die as a result of regular assault by sounds above 85 dB. That's not much noise by today's standards. It's anything louder than a noisy restaurant, a food mixer, or a drive on the highway with the windows down.

Ear injuries

Major traumas, such as skull fractures or concussions, can damage parts of the ear and cause hearing loss, but more common minor traumas can also inflict significant harm. Permanent damage can be done by an ordinary cotton-tipped swab used to clean the outer ear. Sometimes a person simply cleans too deeply. Other times, an accident occurs when someone cleaning his or her ear is bumped or shoved, forcing the cotton swab deep into the ear. Doctors have seen scratched ear canals, torn eardrums, and damaged ossicles caused by cotton swabs.

Changes in air pressure that occur while scuba diving or even flying in an airplane can stretch, bruise, or rupture the eardrum. Scuba diving can also rupture the membranes of the inner ear, allowing fluid to escape. This kind of damage can cause hearing loss and dizziness. It sometimes heals on its own, in which case the symptoms may be temporary. But sometimes the injuries must be surgically repaired, and even surgery doesn't always restore hearing.

Infections

Infections in and around the ear can cause conductive hearing loss. A middle ear infection, or otitis media, is the most common cause of hearing loss in children,

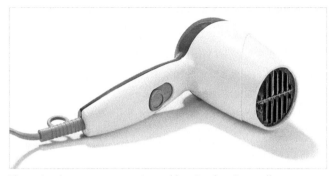

The noise that causes sensorineural hearing loss is usually not one deafening bang but decades' worth of exposure to the high-decibel accessories of daily life: blow dryers, leaf blowers, car horns, traffic, movie theater sounds, and so on.

although adults sometimes get it, too. Such an infection is often accompanied by a buildup of fluid in the middle ear, which hinders sound waves from passing through. The hearing loss is usually temporary, but it can be permanent if infections are recurrent and aren't treated properly.

More common in adults is otitis externa, a bacterial or fungal infection of the skin lining the canal of the outer ear. Otitis externa is also called swimmer's ear because it occurs most often during the summer and tends to affect swimmers and divers. Scratching the outer ear poses an even bigger risk than swimming or diving, since broken skin allows germs to enter and infect the area. The infection can lead to hearing loss by causing a discharge or swelling in the ear canal. Individuals with diabetes or conditions that suppress the immune system, such as HIV infection, are vulnerable to an especially serious kind of otitis externa, which can spread rapidly to the skull or brain.

Another type of infection that can cause hearing loss is labyrinthitis, which affects both the cochlea and the balance organs of the inner ear, leading to hearing loss and dizziness. And meningitis, a brain infection, can damage the auditory nerves.

Be aware that hearing loss that comes on suddenly is sometimes a symptom of an inner ear infection or a blood vessel problem in the inner ear. If you have an abrupt and dramatic loss of hearing, see your doctor immediately. All of these infections are treatable, but you have the best odds of regaining your hearing completely if the problem is diagnosed and you begin treatment a week or less after the onset of the problem.

Otosclerosis

This disorder is the most common cause of conductive hearing loss in young and middle-aged adults. It's characterized by abnormal growth of the bone in the labyrinth of the inner ear. The excess bone can press against the stapes, the smallest of the bones in the middle ear, preventing it from vibrating. Otosclerosis is at least partly genetic. While it runs in families, it can skip several generations, and it's more common in some groups of people than in others. Women are affected more often than men, and Caucasians are more susceptible than African Americans. Hearing aids or surgical repair of the abnormal bone growth can return hearing levels to normal (see "Stapedectomy," page 41).

Medications

Several over-the-counter and prescription drugs can harm the nerves in the inner ear and can cause sudden hearing loss. In many cases, ringing in the ears or vertigo (dizziness) accompanies the hearing loss. With over-the-counter drugs, the problems are usually temporary. In most cases, normal hearing returns and the other symptoms go away several weeks after the medication is stopped. Prescription drugs are more likely to lead to permanent changes in hearing.

Commonly used drugs that can affect hearing include the following:
- aspirin
- aminoglycosides, which include antibiotics such as gentamicin (Garamycin) and amikacin (Amikin)
- cisplatin (Platinol), a chemotherapy drug
- diuretics such as ethacrynic acid (Edecrin) and furosemide (Lasix), which are used for high blood pressure (hypertension)
- quinine (Qualaquin), an antimalaria drug
- quinidine (Cardioquin, Quinidex), a medication for irregular heartbeat
- acetaminophen and hydrocodone (Vicodin), a combination drug prescribed for pain
- PDEs inhibitors (Viagra, Levitra, Cialis), used to treat erectile dysfunction.

Aspirin is a problem only when it's taken too often or in too high a dose. (The low-dose aspirin used for heart disease is fine.) The other drugs implicated in hearing loss can cause adverse reactions in the ear even when taken as directed. If you take one of these drugs and are concerned, ask your doctor if a different drug that doesn't affect hearing is available, especially if you already have some hearing loss.

Earwax

Earwax is a normal, healthy secretion in the outer ear that protects the ear from harmful substances like water, dirt, and germs. But if too much earwax builds up and forms an obstruction (becomes impacted) in the ear canal or around the eardrum, it can cause conductive hearing loss. The problem is more common with age because earwax becomes drier, and the drier it is, the more likely it is to become impacted.

The tendency to have dry earwax is also inherited; one study published in *Nature Genetics* linked it to a variant of the ABCC11 gene. But regardless of your age and genetic profile, anything that pushes earwax down the ear canal can impair hearing. For example, while cleaning earwax from the outer ear, you may inadvertently push some deeper into the ear. Sometimes wearing a hearing aid causes the problem by forcing earwax from the outer ear deeper into the ear canal. In addition to interfering with hearing, a buildup of earwax often causes discomfort or a feeling of pressure in the ear.

Genetics

Hearing loss runs in families. If one or both of your parents became deaf in their advanced years, you have a higher-than-average chance of age-related hearing loss. Research has identified several genes linked to hearing. Some of these genes affect the production and function of sensory hair cells. For example, mutations in the transmembrane cochlear-expressed gene are the cause of deafness in two-thirds of people with hereditary hearing loss.

Genetic testing is not recommended because it is expensive, it is not typically covered by insurance, and the results do not have any impact on how hearing loss is treated. Genetic tests are more commonly performed on newborns who are deaf or hard of hearing. The tests provide information about the child's hearing loss that can help prepare parents for what to expect over the course of time. They can also predict

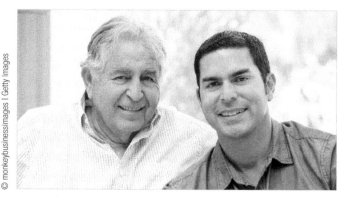

Hearing loss within a family may be the result of shared genes. Multiple genetic mutations are known to cause hearing loss. But there are many other causes as well, such as infections.

the chances that future children will have a hearing problem. In children, hearing impairment sometimes results from disorders caused by genetic defects that interfered with the development of their hearing mechanism before birth. Such disorders include Waardenburg syndrome and Usher's syndrome. In addition, some chromosomal abnormalities, such as Down syndrome, can cause hearing loss.

Congenital problems

The word congenital means "born with." But congenital problems aren't necessarily genetic. Various complications during pregnancy can impair the development of hearing in the fetus. These complications include infection with herpes, syphilis, or cytomegalovirus (a virus that is related to herpes), as well as the use of medications, such as quinine, that can damage the hearing mechanism. In addition, premature birth increases the risk of hearing loss in babies and young children.

Ménière's disease

This disorder, which interferes with balance and hearing, affects about 615,000 people in the United States, mainly women over 40, and another 45,500 are diagnosed each year. Its cause is unknown. Doctors have long thought that some cases are triggered by migraines. Another likely cause is damage from an inner ear infection. Unlike many other causes of hearing loss, which lead to constant difficulty hearing, Ménière's causes spells of hearing loss that come and go. These spells are accompanied by episodes of vertigo and tinnitus. One or both ears may be affected.

Ménière's symptoms are caused by an accumulation of endolymph, a kind of fluid in the inner ear. The fluid builds up to the point that the membranes that contain it rupture, damaging the sensory cells around them. An attack of Ménière's can last minutes or hours. Afterward, the dizziness and tinnitus stop and hearing usually returns to normal. But with each attack, persistent tinnitus and hearing loss become more likely.

No two people with Ménière's have the same experience. Some get just one attack in their lives; others have a second attack many years later; still others have attacks every month or even every day. Sometimes the condition stops on its own, but in other cases sufferers need medication or surgery for relief.

Tumors

Several kinds of benign or malignant tumors can grow in the ear and cause hearing loss, tinnitus, and dizziness.

Acoustic neuroma. A benign growth on the balance nerve in the inner ear, acoustic neuroma is the most common type of nerve tumor affecting this area. About one in 100,000 people per year develops the problem. It affects mostly Caucasians and usually appears between the ages of 50 and 64. An acoustic neuroma usually makes itself known with hearing loss resulting from pressure on the auditory nerve. Although it is not malignant, an acoustic neuroma can cause serious problems or death if it becomes big enough to press on the brain. Treatment options include surgery or radiation. The decision over which option is best depends on the size of the tumor and the age of the patient. Most small tumors are simply observed initially, because many will never grow.

Glomus tympanicum and glomus jugulare. These are benign growths in the blood vessels of the ear. In addition to hearing loss, these tumors often cause a pulsing ringing in the ears. As with acoustic neuromas, glomus tumors need to be observed regularly by a doctor. If they grow too big, they must be shrunk with radiation or removed surgically.

Cholesteatoma. Yet another benign growth that can cause hearing loss is a cholesteatoma, or a cyst in the middle ear. As it grows, the cyst can harm the middle ear, causing conductive hearing loss. If it gets big enough to enter the inner ear, it can lead to sensorineural hearing loss as well. Cholesteatomas are usually surgically removed.

Malignant tumors. Although far less common than the benign tumors, certain forms of cancer can also impair hearing. These include cancers of the ear and the brain, as well as cancer in other parts of the body (such as the breast, lung, or kidney) that spreads to the temporal bone of the skull, which contains the ear.

Other causes

Hearing loss is sometimes a side effect of certain illnesses. Autoimmune diseases, in which a person's immune system goes awry and attacks his or her own body, can cause hearing loss if the immune system attacks the ear tissue. Autoimmune diseases include lupus, multiple sclerosis, and autoimmune inner ear disease, the rare condition that caused rapid and profound hearing loss in Rush Limbaugh, the radio talk-show host, in 2001. Limbaugh's hearing was restored through a cochlear implant. In addition, people who had many ear infections as children may have permanent holes in their eardrums. The holes can cause conductive hearing loss by interfering with the eardrum's functioning.

Hearing loss and brain health

Hearing loss is often believed to be more of a nuisance than a condition that affects overall health. But within the past decade, scientists have found an interesting association between hearing loss and problems with brain function.

In a 2013 study of 1,984 older adults who were living independently and followed for 11 years, researchers found that hearing loss is independently associated with accelerated cognitive decline. Those participants who had hearing loss at the outset of the study had a 24% increased risk for cognitive impairment compared with those who had normal hearing. The study, published in *JAMA Internal Medicine*, pointed out that more studies are needed to explain the association. Researchers are also looking into whether treatment with hearing aids would protect the brain from decline.

A smaller study produced similar findings in 2012. Researchers at Johns Hopkins University followed a group of 639 older adults for an average of 11.9 years and found that those with mild hearing loss at the outset had twice the risk of developing dementia by the end; those with moderate hearing loss had three times the risk, and those with severe hearing loss had five times the risk. The reasons for this pattern are not yet known.

One possibility, suggested by the researchers in both studies, is that when people struggle with their hearing, they often withdraw from social interactions with family and friends. Not only does such withdrawal lead to depression, but the isolation in itself is a known risk factor for dementia.

Another study, this one from the University of Pennsylvania, took a different approach. This time researchers used brain scans to measure the relationship between hearing acuity and brain volume in a group of adults ages 60 to 77. The study found that people with hearing loss had less gray matter in the auditory cortex (the area of the brain that makes sense out of the sounds you hear). They also showed less brain activity on functional MRI scans when listening to a series of increasingly complex sentences. The researchers hypothesized that a decline in hearing accelerates a decline in brain function in areas related to auditory processing, with "cascading consequences" for neural processes that support perception and cognition.

That said, it is still too soon to conclude that hearing loss is an independent risk factor for dementia. In 2017, researchers reviewed 17 such studies and found flaws in a number of them. For example, some of the studies did not control for other risk factors for dementia. In others, hearing loss itself could have explained why individuals did not perform well on the cognitive tests. The authors of the review, published in *Laryngoscope Investigative Otolaryngology*, concluded that the research has provided valuable insight into the correlation between hearing loss and dementia. However, more research is needed to determine if there is a direct causal relationship between hearing loss and cognitive decline.

Either way, it is safe to assume that social isolation can contribute to depression and cognitive decline, and it is clear that treating hearing loss is essential to preserving one's ability to communicate and stay connected.

Testing for hearing loss

Given that hearing loss usually occurs gradually, it can take years for a person to accept the fact that he or she needs a hearing evaluation. Many people remain unconvinced of the problem as long as they can compensate by asking others to repeat what they've said or by turning up the TV or phone volume. Some think there's little point to seeing a doctor until these means of compensation no longer work. When people finally do take action, it's often at the suggestion of close relatives or friends who are exasperated with the constant need to repeat themselves.

Having your hearing "checked" is actually a multistep process that can involve two health practitioners: a doctor and an audiologist (someone who specializes in testing for hearing loss and fitting hearing aids). If you suspect that you're losing your hearing, first see a doctor who specializes in hearing disorders (see "The hearing professionals," above right).

The medical exam

Two medical specialties are devoted to hearing. Otolaryngologists focus on problems of the ears as well as the nose and throat, and are therefore commonly called "ear, nose, and throat doctors." Otologists specialize exclusively in ear problems. Either of these specialists can perform a physical exam and some general hearing tests to determine the cause of your hearing loss and narrow down the list of possible solutions. Your primary care physician may also do preliminary hearing loss screening, described in this section, before referring you to a specialist.

The physical exam for hearing loss consists mainly of questions regarding your medical history. Be prepared for the doctor to ask you a lot of questions. For example, how long have you had trouble hearing? Did the problem come on gradually or suddenly? In what situations do you have the most difficulty hearing? Age-related hearing loss typically comes on over a period of years, but hearing loss that occurs suddenly may be caused by an infection or a medication you've recently started taking.

There are other important questions. Is the hearing loss in one or both ears? With age, the hearing in both ears usually declines at roughly the same rate (although one ear might be stronger than the other). Hearing loss that is far worse in one ear suggests a medical problem, such as an ear infection, an injury, a blockage of earwax, or an abnormal growth. Are there other symptoms, such as ringing in the ears or dizziness? While ringing in the ears often occurs along with age-related hearing loss, it can also be a sign of other problems, including Ménière's disease (see page 11), an ear infec-

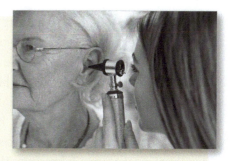

The hearing professionals

Chances are, you will see more than one health professional to help diagnose and treat your hearing loss. Here is a guide to hearing loss professionals and their fields of expertise.

Otolaryngologists. Also called "ear, nose, and throat doctors," or ENTs, these specialists perform medical evaluations and basic hearing tests. ENTs also perform surgery on the ear to treat hearing loss and related conditions, such as dizziness.

Otologists. These are doctors who specialize in treating ear problems. Otologists and otolaryngologists are equally qualified to diagnose and treat hearing problems, including performing surgery on the ear.

Audiologists. These are professionals trained to perform hearing evaluations, interpret the results, diagnose certain ear disorders, make proper referrals, and fit hearing aids. Audiologists have at least a master's degree. Some have a state license to dispense hearing aids.

tion (see "Infections," page 9), or even nerve damage from a medication (see "Medications," page 10).

The doctor will also ask about the particular situations in which you have the most difficulty hearing. For example, do you have trouble hearing in places where a lot of people are talking at once? This suggests hearing loss in the high-frequency range, the typical pattern that occurs with age. Do you struggle to hear all conversations, even one-on-one conversations in a quiet room? That indicates severe hearing loss.

As part of your evaluation, the doctor will also ask about your general health history, because some conditions, such as head injuries, chronic ear infections, or allergies, can impair hearing. The doctor may ask you about your occupation and hobbies. Those that involve exposure to loud noises—like construction work, hunting, or playing a loud musical instrument—can cause sensorineural hearing loss by degrading the hair cells in the inner ear.

Finally, the doctor examines your ears, as well as your throat, mouth, and nose, since infections or growths in these areas can impair hearing. The doctor looks into your ears with an otoscope (an instrument that shines a bright light) to illuminate physical abnormalities that can affect hearing, such as blockages or growths in the ear canal, inflammation or perforation of the eardrum, and fluid behind the eardrum. If you have an ear infection, the doctor will give you antibiotics to cure it. If there's no improvement, you'll need to have your hearing tested.

For most people, the centerpiece of the diagnostic process is a series of tests to determine the severity of the hearing loss and the range of frequencies where it occurs. The physician performs only the most basic of these tests—the Weber test and the Rinne test. They take just a few minutes and aren't uncomfortable at all. Both tests involve using a tuning fork that sends vibrations into the ear to help assess whether your hearing loss is conductive, sensorineural, or both.

Weber test

This test reveals whether your hearing is stronger in one ear than in the other. The doctor first makes the tuning fork vibrate by striking it against a hard surface, then holds the stem of the fork against the center of your forehead. The vibrations are transmitted through the bone directly to the inner ear to produce audible sound. The doctor will ask you to identify the ear in which the vibrations seem louder. If you can't hear a difference, both ears have roughly equal hearing capacity. If the sound is louder in one ear, that can mean one of two things. There may be sensorineural hearing loss in the ear where the sound is fainter, because the nerves can't respond to the vibrations. Or, counterintuitively, there may be conductive hearing loss in the ear where the sound is louder, because the vibrations are bypassing an obstruction in the middle ear. (In that case, the tuning fork would sound louder because it would not have to compete for attention with ambient sounds, which would have trouble passing through a middle ear obstruction.)

Rinne test

To figure out which kind of hearing loss you have, the doctor will perform a Rinne test. This two-part test compares how well you hear sound that travels by air through the outer and middle ear with how well you hear sound that's conducted directly through the mastoid bone to the inner ear. For the air-conduction part of the test, the doctor holds the vibrating tuning fork a few inches away from each ear. For the bone-conduction part of the test, the doctor holds the base of the vibrating tuning fork against the mastoid bone behind the ear. Then, the doctor asks you whether the tone of the vibrating fork was louder during the first or second part of the test. If the middle ear is working normally, the sound will be louder by air conduction. When the sound is louder by the bone, the ear has conductive hearing loss. By combining the Rinne and Weber tests, a doctor can evaluate the presence of an asymmetrical hearing loss.

It's important to note that someone with symmetrical hearing loss (the same level of sensorineural hearing loss in both ears) can still have normal Rinne and Weber tests.

To make the Rinne test as accurate as possible, the doctor creates "white noise" outside the ear that isn't being tested. The purpose is to keep that ear from picking up some of the sound intended for the ear being tested, possibly compensating for some of the tested ear's hearing loss. Many people with severe hearing loss in one ear can compensate reasonably well by hearing sounds in their better ear. This compensation is entirely unconscious—sometimes, the brain actually shifts the perception of incoming sounds, a phenomenon called interaural attenuation. The white noise distracts the ear not being tested so that it doesn't hear the test sounds.

Audioscope testing

In their role as primary care physicians, some internists and pediatricians do another hearing test to screen for hearing loss using an audioscope, a handheld device, to play tones into each ear. The tones are of different frequencies, usually set at 40 decibels (dB), which is the volume of normal speech. People who can't hear sounds at this decibel level usually need a hearing aid. By identifying which of these frequencies you can hear and which ones you can't, the doctor can tell the frequency range where your hearing loss is concentrated and then make specific recommendations for more refined hearing tests by an audiologist.

The audiological evaluation

If the doctor's preliminary testing confirms your suspicion that your hearing is impaired, then you'll be referred for an audiological evaluation, an extensive battery of tests performed by an audiologist. An audiological evaluation identifies the type of hearing loss (sensorineural, conductive, or mixed), how severe it is (see Table 1, above right), and the frequency range in which it occurs. This information may help your doctor diagnose the cause of your hearing loss. It's also essential for determining whether you could benefit from a hearing aid and, if so, which style and type of circuitry would help the most. Chances are that your doctor works with an audiologist or can recommend one to you.

The series of hearing tests performed by an audiologist usually takes about 20 to 30 minutes. This round of tests is done in a specially constructed, soundproof booth in order to shut out unwanted noise and ensure accurate results. You'll listen to sounds through each ear separately while wearing earphones. The audiologist generates the sounds using a control panel in an adjoining booth. You'll probably be able to see the audiologist through a window, and you'll be able to speak with him or her at any time during the evaluation. The audiologist will do more than one kind of test. One is a pure-tone test, which identifies the quietest tones that you can hear in low, mid-range, and high frequencies. Additional testing evaluates how well you hear and understand spoken words.

Table 1: Degrees of hearing loss

Hearing loss is measured on a scale from mild to profound, according to the softest sound that you can hear in a particular frequency range. The softest sounds and their corresponding rankings are shown below. To determine the severity of your hearing loss in each frequency range, your audiologist and doctor will evaluate your audiogram against this chart. If, for example, the softest sound you can hear in the low-frequency range is 65 decibels (dB), you have moderately severe hearing loss in that range. Keep in mind it's possible to have normal hearing in the low frequencies but moderate or severe hearing loss in the high-frequency range.

LOWEST VOLUME AUDIBLE	HEARING LOSS CATEGORY
0–25 dB	Normal hearing
26–40 dB	Mild hearing loss
41–55 dB	Moderate hearing loss
56–69 dB	Moderately severe hearing loss
70–90 dB	Severe hearing loss
91 dB and above	Profound hearing loss

Pure-tone testing

For this test, the audiologist uses an electronic machine called an audiometer to expose each ear, in turn, to sounds of different frequencies and decibel levels. The purpose is to identify the frequencies at which you have trouble hearing and how much hearing loss you have in those frequencies—in other words, how difficult it is for you to hear high-pitched or low-pitched sounds, or both.

The audiologist will probably start with middle-frequency tones of 1,000 Hz and then gradually go up to high-frequency tones of 8,000 Hz, and finally test the low-frequency tones down to 250 Hz. The range of tones tested is roughly equivalent to a span of low to high notes on a piano. After identifying the lowest decibel level at which you can hear a tone of a certain frequency, the audiologist moves on to another frequency tone. The results are plotted on an audiogram, a graph that shows how well each ear hears across the frequency spectrum. This graph is as individual as a signature—it's your personal pattern of hearing (see Figure 4, at right).

People with normal hearing can hear tones of 25 dB or less across the frequency (pitch) spectrum. But your audiogram might show, for example, that your right ear has normal hearing at low frequencies up to 1,000 Hz, but that it can't hear high-pitched tones softer than 60 dB at 2,000 Hz, an indication of moderate hearing loss at that frequency. In that case, the audiologist will want to pinpoint the frequency at which the hearing loss in your right ear begins. To do that, the audiologist tests your ability to hear tones of, say, 1,500 Hz and then, depending on what's found, works up or down from there. The same kind of testing is done on your left ear.

Next, the audiologist does a bone-conduction test to compare how well you hear sounds that are routed directly to the nerves in the inner ear with how well you just heard the tones through the earphones. To do this, the audiologist places a vibrating tool, called a bone oscillator, on the bone behind the ear. The vibrations travel through the mastoid bone in the skull behind the ear to the nerves in the inner ear. The result of the bone-conduction test compared with the result of the pure-tone test indicates whether your hearing loss is primarily sensorineural or conductive, or a combination of the two. It will also help determine whether you have a medically correctable form of hearing loss and the kind of hearing aid you need.

If the bone-conduction levels match the levels of the tones that you hear through headphones and you have hearing loss, the problem is mainly sensorineural. This result indicates that the middle ear is working properly. But if you can hear tones better with the bone-conduction test, the problem is mainly conductive. In other words, there is a structural problem with the eardrum or the ossicles in the middle ear. The results of the bone-conduction and pure-tone tests are put on the audiogram.

Interpreting your audiogram. To understand your audiogram, look first at the frequency range

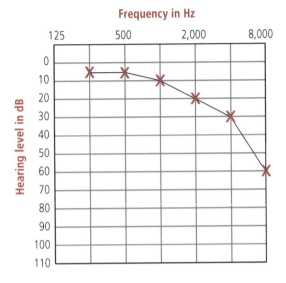

Figure 4: Understanding your audiogram

An audiogram tells you how well you hear sounds of increasing frequency (pitch). The decibel level (vertical axis) represents the loudness required for you to hear the sound at each frequency. In this example (which shows results from the left ear), the person's hearing decreases as the frequency of the sound increases. In other words, this person demonstrates a typical pattern of age-associated hearing loss (presbycusis), in which higher-pitch sounds are more difficult to hear. People with normal hearing can hear tones of 25 dB or less across the frequency spectrum.

(pitch) shown from left to right (see Figure 4, above); the lowest sounds are on the left. The decibel levels (loudness) are shown from top to bottom, with the quietest sounds at the top. Hearing in the left ear is plotted as a line connecting X's on the graph, the right ear as connecting O's. (Figure 4 shows the results from a left-ear audiogram only.) The pattern of the hearing lines on the audiogram indicates the nature and severity of your hearing loss. Normal hearing appears as two flat lines close to the top, at or above 25 dB. The closer to the bottom the lines fall, the weaker your hearing is. If the lines representing each ear overlap or are close together, the hearing ability of both ears is similar, whereas if one line is closer to the top, the ear that it represents is the stronger one.

The pattern of the lines on the audiogram also reveals information about the nature of your hearing. Flat lines indicate that your hearing is the same across the frequency ranges, but lines that go up and down show that your hearing is better in some frequencies than others. Age-related hearing loss (presbycusis) tends to look like the right half of a mountain: the lines start out high, then plunge steadily. This means that hearing is normal at low frequencies but drops off in the middle and high frequencies. Exactly where this drop occurs and how low it goes varies from one person to the next. Unfortunately, speech falls mainly in the middle and high frequencies, and background noises—such as the din of a restaurant or other crowded space—tend to be in the low frequencies. For people with presbycusis, this means conversations are not only harder to hear than they used to be, but also increasingly drowned out by background noise.

The shape of the pure-tone test results on the audiogram can only estimate the difficulty you may have hearing someone speak in real-life situations. To assess your ability to hear words clearly, the audiologist will perform two more tests.

Speech reception threshold
Hearing tones is one thing; understanding spoken words is another. Strange as it may seem, it is possible to practically ace the pure-tone test by hearing sounds at 25 dB in many frequencies, but still not be able to understand words spoken at that decibel level. The speech reception test identifies the lowest decibel level at which you can understand at least half the words spoken. For this test, you sit in the soundproof booth with earphones on, but you hear words, instead of tones, through your earphones. An audiologist or someone on a recording speaks simple two-syllable words. The audiologist asks you to repeat the words you hear. The words start out fairly loud and then gradually get softer and softer. The softer they get, the fewer of them you'll be able to understand and repeat accurately. The test is over when the audiologist has found the decibel level at which you can understand and repeat only half of the words.

Speech discrimination
Everyone has had this experience: someone is talking to you, and you can hear the words loudly but not clearly. The problem is especially common when you're trying to have a conversation in a noisy room. With age, however, many people have this problem even in quiet settings. The words are loud, but they sound garbled.

A speech discrimination test assesses how well you understand words. For this test, the audiologist has you listen to words through the headphones at a decibel level louder than your speech reception threshold, so you won't have any problem with the volume of the speech. This test uses one-syllable words with vowels and consonants that are distributed similarly to those of words used in ordinary conversations—words such as "jar," "this," and "box." The audiologist asks you to repeat the words you hear. Successfully repeating 90% or more of them is considered excellent.

Although it doesn't mean your hearing is good, a high score on the speech discrimination test is good news. It means that you stand to benefit the most from a hearing aid, because boosting the volume of words will help you understand them better. In other words, your problem is mainly volume, which a hearing aid can help. If you understand only a low percentage of the words, simply turning up the volume with a hearing aid is unlikely to help you hear any more clearly.

The main cause of difficulty with word discrimination is inner-ear hair cell or nerve degeneration. If your trouble understanding words is modest, a hearing aid may help to some degree, but it will not fully remedy the problem. You'll still need to use visual cues, such as lip reading, to help you understand what a person is saying. The more severe your problem is with word discrimination, the more limited your benefit from using a hearing aid.

Other hearing tests
The tests listed above make up the standard audiological exam, but depending on the results, other tests may be needed.

Tympanometry. The most common additional test is tympanometry, or impedance testing, which is done if your audiological exam suggests that your hearing difficulty is in the middle ear. For this test, an earplug attached to a machine called a tympanometer is placed in the ear. Tones and air pressure are channeled through the plug into the ear canal to make the eardrum move. The tympanometer then records the eardrum's movement. No movement, or less movement than normal, indicates that there is a middle ear problem, such as fluid in the middle ear. The audiologist will refer you to an otolaryngologist or otologist for a diagnosis.

Acoustic reflex threshold testing. Although it's not new, this test is being used more frequently because of a growing recognition that it's helpful in diagnosing problems beyond the inner ear, in the pathways leading to the brain. The purpose of the test is to see if the ear's natural reflex to lower the volume of very loud sounds is working properly. The test is conducted like tympanometry, but in addition to using the pressurized probe, the audiologist delivers a sound of about 80 dB to see if the muscles in the middle ear contract to decrease the volume. The audiologist keeps increasing or decreasing the volume to find the decibel level at which this reflex occurs. It normally occurs at 65 to 95 dB. A reflex that starts at a higher decibel level or doesn't occur at all suggests that your hearing loss may be at least partially the result of a neurological problem.

Otoacoustic emissions test. This test assesses whether the hair cells of the cochlea, in the inner ear, are functioning. Normally, hair cells emit sound in response to incoming sounds. Otoacoustic testing detects the hair cell sound with a rubber-tipped probe inserted into the ear canal. The procedure usually takes less than five minutes for each ear. The absence of sound from the hair cells can mean either a problem with the cochlea or mild conductive hearing loss. The test is used, sometimes in combination with the evoked potential test (see page 19), to screen babies before they leave the hospital and is also used in young children, meaning doctors can now identify

Do-it-yourself, five-minute hearing test

This questionnaire can help you evaluate the severity of your hearing loss. Write the number of points next to the answer that best describes your hearing.

1. I have a problem hearing over the telephone. ____
   Almost always (3)
   Half of the time (2)
   Occasionally (1)
   Never (0)

2. I have trouble following the conversation when two or more people are talking at the same time. ____
   Almost always (3)
   Half of the time (2)
   Occasionally (1)
   Never (0)

3. People complain that I turn the television volume up too high. ____
   Almost always (3)
   Half of the time (2)
   Occasionally (1)
   Never (0)

4. I have to strain to understand conversations. ____
   Almost always (3)
   Half of the time (2)
   Occasionally (1)
   Never (0)

5. I miss hearing some common sounds like the phone or doorbell ringing. ____
   Almost always (3)
   Half of the time (2)
   Occasionally (1)
   Never (0)

6. I have trouble hearing conversations in a noisy background, such as at a party. ____
   Almost always (3)
   Half of the time (2)
   Occasionally (1)
   Never (0)

7. I get confused about where sounds come from. ____
   Almost always (3)
   Half of the time (2)
   Occasionally (1)
   Never (0)

8. I misunderstand some words in a sentence and need to ask people to repeat themselves. ____
   Almost always (3)
   Half of the time (2)
   Occasionally (1)
   Never (0)

a child's hearing loss much earlier than in years past. The otoacoustic test is also becoming increasingly common for adults who have sensorineural hearing loss or tinnitus or who are taking medications that can damage the ear.

Evoked potential test. This test may be done either if the results of your audiogram are unclear or if the hearing in one ear is significantly worse than the hearing in the other. Your doctor or audiologist may also call this an auditory brainstem response test or an auditory evoked response test.

This test measures how the auditory nerve and the brain respond to sound. It takes about half an hour and is more involved than the other tests. You lie down with earphones on, and the audiologist places electrodes on your ears, forehead, and the top of your head. The electrode wires are attached to a computer. A repetitive, loud clicking sound is played through the headphones to one ear at a time, and the computer measures the electrical response to the sound by the nerves of the ear and brainstem.

Two qualities of this response are important: timing and strength. Both should be within normal limits based on an established standard, and they should also be similar in both ears. An asymmetry, a delayed response, or a weak response indicates that an illness or an abnormality is affecting the auditory pathway.

Imaging tests. If the evoked potential test is inconclusive, your doctor might order an imaging test, either a CT scan or an MRI, to look for abnormal growths in the ears or the brain. The doctor may order one of these tests without first asking for an evoked potential test if your medical history seems to indicate a tumor as the cause of your hearing loss.

---

9. I especially have trouble understanding the speech of women and children. ____
   Almost always (3)
   Half of the time (2)
   Occasionally (1)
   Never (0)

10. I have worked in noisy environments (assembly line, construction site, airport runway, etc.). ____
    Almost always (3)
    Half of the time (2)
    Occasionally (1)
    Never (0)

11. Many people I talk to seem to mumble (or don't speak clearly). ____
    Almost always (3)
    Half of the time (2)
    Occasionally (1)
    Never (0)

12. People get annoyed because I misunderstand what they say. ____
    Almost always (3)
    Half of the time (2)
    Occasionally (1)
    Never (0)

13. I misunderstand what others are saying and respond inappropriately. ____
    Almost always (3)
    Half of the time (2)
    Occasionally (1)
    Never (0)

14. I avoid social activities because I cannot hear well and fear I'll reply improperly. ____
    Almost always (3)
    Half of the time (2)
    Occasionally (1)
    Never (0)

To be answered by a family member or friend:

15. Do you think this person has hearing loss? ____
    Almost always (3)
    Half of the time (2)
    Occasionally (1)
    Never (0)

> **SCORING**
> Add your total points. A score below 6 indicates no problem with your hearing. A score of 6 to 9 is in the middle range, indicating that a hearing check-up is advisable. A score of 10 or above indicates that a visit to a medical hearing professional is strongly advised.

Adapted with permission from the American Academy of Otolaryngology–Head and Neck Surgery.

SPECIAL SECTION

Selecting a hearing aid

Like cellphones, computers, and televisions, hearing technology has benefited from the digital revolution. As a result, hearing aids are smaller and have better sound quality than ever before. And this quality continues to improve with each passing year, on pace with improvements in the audio technology in smartphones, portable speakers, and headphones. As the technology continues to evolve, hearing aids have gained new capabilities. Today even the most basic hearing aids offer wireless technology, including connectivity to cellphones, televisions, and digital music players.

Every year, new models are introduced with new features and new variations on old features. Just as buying a television set has changed from a simple matter to a head-spinning experience with a multitude of choices, so too has the task of finding the right hearing device become more complicated. This chapter contains a step-by-step guide to choosing the right one for your lifestyle and needs.

Hearing aids then and now

Hearing aids have changed considerably over time. So, if you're thinking about the bulky, unattractive hearing aids people wore years ago, you're in for a pleasant surprise. There are many choices now in size, shape, price, and type of technology (see Figure 5, page 21). Newer hearing aids are smaller and produce better sound quality with less distortion than those of the past.

From trumpet to transistor

Instruments to aid hearing have been around for more than 300 years. Originally, they were just tubes and trumpets that people held to their ears to amplify incoming sound. The first electrical hearing aids were built near the end of the 19th century. They consisted of an earphone connected to a microphone that was attached to a battery box. One hearing aid pioneer was Alexander Graham Bell, who built the first earphone to amplify sound for people who were hard of hearing.

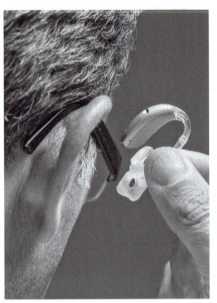

Hearing aids have better sound quality than ever before. Every year new models are introduced with new features and new variations on old features.

Until the 1950s, there was just one kind of hearing aid—a cumbersome box that you strapped to your body. It had a thick wire that snaked up to an earpiece that fit into the opening of the ear. Today, there are hundreds of different models of hearing aids and dozens of manufacturers.

The digital revolution

The advent of digital sound processing was a major advance in improving the quality of sound

Selecting a hearing aid | **SPECIAL SECTION**

produced by hearing aids. Unlike the analog hearing aids that came before them, digital hearing aids do not treat all sounds the same. Instead, they selectively amplify, emphasizing speech sounds and de-emphasizing noise (see "Choosing circuitry," page 31). Digital technology also enables the hearing aid to automatically adjust itself to changing environments, eliminating the need for volume control.

Even with their impressive advances, all hearing aids have the same primary purpose: to amplify the sounds you want to hear. They have the same basic components, and most run on batteries. They contain at least one microphone that picks up sound and converts it into electrical signals. These signals are transmitted to an amplifier, which boosts their strength and alters the sounds. The amplified electrical signals then travel to a receiver, a small loudspeaker that converts the electrical signals back into sound waves and channels them into the ear. The hearing aids of more than a hundred years ago amplified sounds by only a few decibels, making little practical difference in what a person could hear. By contrast, the hearing aids of today can boost sound by as much as 80 dB or more. That's roughly the difference between a whisper and a car horn.

With such powerful amplification, it's only natural to wonder if hearing aids can further deteriorate hearing. The answer is yes, if their maximum volume is set too high. That's why it's extremely important to find a reputable hearing aid professional, often called a dispenser, who will adjust the volume properly so it's loud enough to meet your needs but not so loud as to be harmful.

You can add to the basic components to improve a hearing aid's sound quality. Optional digital circuitry is available to help reduce unwanted background noise, for example, or to enhance the quality of musical sounds or improve sound over the telephone.

Another category of hearing devices is known as assistive listening devices. This term refers to a wide variety of devices that are used in addition to or instead of hearing aids to help you hear, using Bluetooth transmission to stream sound, in some cases, directly to your hearing aids. Most are situational—that is, you use them in situations in which you have difficulty. For instance, there are listening systems for TVs, radios, or stereos that minimize interference from surrounding noise and amplify the desired sound for the listener. Hearing aid–compatible phones allow hearing aids to be used at a comfortable volume with minimal feedback. Other examples include personal listening systems that help with interpersonal conversation in noisy locations, wireless connectivity to cellphones, and

Figure 5: Shapes and sizes of hearing aids

The variety of hearing aid choices continues to grow. Shown here from left to right: completely-in-the-canal (CIC), in-the-canal (ITC), in-the-ear (ITE), standard behind-the-ear (BTE), rechargeable BTE, receiver-in-the-canal (RIC) BTE, invisible-in-the-canal (IIC), and Lyric extended-wear.

Completely-in-the-canal

In-the-canal

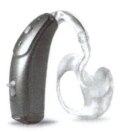
In-the-ear

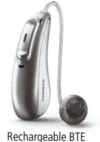
Behind-the-ear

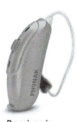
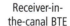
Rechargeable BTE

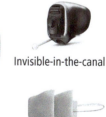
Receiver-in-the-canal BTE

Invisible-in-the-canal

Lyric extended-wear

Behind-the-ear photo by Mark Stockwell. All others courtesy of Phonak.

SPECIAL SECTION | Selecting a hearing aid

alerting devices that flash a light, for example, when the phone or doorbell rings.

Wireless connectivity

With advances in wireless technology, certain hearing aids are now capable of sending signals back and forth from one to the other so that both ears can process sound together. Changes in programming and use of volume adjustments can be made to both ears by using only one program button. This technology has improved tremendously in just the past few years, enhancing the quality and clarity of sound.

In addition, most manufacturers offer hearing aids capable of wireless connections to TVs, cellphones, landline phones, digital music players, and other audio devices. With a wireless connection, you don't have to hold the phone to your ear to hear the person on the other end of the line. If you're watching TV, you can leave the room and come back, and your hearing aids will automatically be reconnected to the sound.

Wireless connection requires a unit that serves as an interface to pick up the signal from compatible devices and transmit it to the hearing aid (see "Wireless interfaces," page 25). Initially, all of these devices used Bluetooth as the interface, and the listener had to wear the Bluetooth unit around his or her neck. Now some companies, such as Starkey, Resound, and Phonak, have developed wireless systems that don't require Bluetooth, so the interface can simply be placed near the audio device you want to hear. This means your hands are free and you don't have to wear anything. With certain hearing aids and the right app, your smartphone can even serve as the interface (see "There's an app for that," at left). But wireless technology takes up space in a hearing aid, so it is more commonly offered in the larger behind-the-ear and in-the-ear models.

Before you buy your hearing aids

One of the most confusing things about deciding which hearing aid to buy is distinguishing the terms that describe style (in-the-ear, behind-the-ear, etc.) from the terms that describe the circuitry inside (digital, programmable, etc.). The hearing aid style and circuitry that you choose depend on many things, including the following:

The nature of your hearing loss. Depending on the specifics of your hearing loss, including its cause and severity and the find-

---

There's an app for that

If you carry a smartphone, you are likely to be able to use it to control your hearing aids. Both the TruLink Hearing Control app from Starkey and the Resound Smart app from Resound allow you to use your phone to wirelessly adjust volume and frequency (treble, bass, etc.) to suit your surroundings. For instance, you can go into a restaurant, adjust your hearing aids to your liking, and geotag the restaurant. Then, when you return to that location, the app will ask you if you want to restore the settings you used the last time you were there. You can create different settings for the different venues you routinely encounter, whether a restaurant, a conference room, an auditorium, or a library.

Yet another app, the Thrive Hearing Control app, enables you to track movement, the number of steps you take, and vital signs such as your heart rate, as sensed by your hearing aids. In addition, the app monitors whether you've had conversations with others that day, in order to help prevent social isolation, and it can even send alerts to selected contacts if you fall. It is compatible with Livio AI hearing aids, manufactured by Starkey, that have built-in sensors and artificial intelligence. Since studies show that people who track their health activities are more motivated to stay healthy, the hearing aid was developed to help facilitate not only improved hearing but staying active.

Hearing aid–compatible apps enable you to manipulate your hearing aid settings easily and unobtrusively. With smartphone use so common in public, you won't necessarily draw attention to yourself when adjusting your settings.

In addition, the apps enable your phone to serve as an assisted listening device so that you can stream phone calls, music, and videos directly to your ears from your cellphone or tablet. The apps, which are available on iTunes or Google Play Store, work only with smartphone-compatible hearing aids.

ings of your audiogram, your audiologist or hearing instrument specialist will make certain recommendations. For example, if you have severe hearing loss, you may need one of the larger hearing aids. Although this is gradually changing, small hearing aids are typically too small to contain circuitry powerful enough to help someone with more than moderately severe hearing loss.

Even if you have mild or moderate hearing loss, the smallest hearing aids may not be the best choice for you. If you are prone to an excessive buildup of earwax or to ear infections, for example, small hearing aids may be easily damaged by earwax or draining ear fluid. Finally, you may want the capability to reduce some types of background noise and boost the sound frequencies you have the most trouble hearing; these optional features are not always available in very small hearing aids.

Your lifestyle. How comfortable are you using wireless devices? This is an important consideration when choosing a hearing aid. If you use electronic devices like cellphones, music players, or laptops that are capable of sending a wireless signal, then you may want your hearing aids to be set up for wireless connection, both with each other and with the devices you use.

You should also consider the demands you will be placing on a hearing aid. If you have a job or a social life that involves a lot of meetings, social engagements, or phone calls, you may require the enhanced features of a premium-technology hearing aid. On the other hand, if you stick close to home, work in a quiet office, and don't frequent many different kinds of acoustic environments, entry-level technology may provide enough noticeable improvement.

Appearance. Keep in mind that the audiologist's recommendations will be based first and foremost on the devices that will provide you with the best hearing. But there will be other considerations, such as how the hearing aid looks. If the cosmetic factor is a concern to you, be sure to let your audiologist know, and he or she will help you narrow down the choices to what will best suit both your hearing needs and your appearance concerns.

Cost. Another factor is cost—hearing aids range in price from about $1,400 to $3,700 each, depending on their size and features. Most of this cost must be paid out of pocket because Medicare and most other insurance plans don't cover hearing aids. (Some Medicare Advantage plans give partial payment.) Always check with your carrier.

Your dexterity. Finally, consider your skill at handling small objects. If you have arthritis, for instance, you may find it difficult to insert and remove the smallest hearing aids and gladly opt for a larger model that's easier to handle.

Will it sound the same?

Be aware that although hearing aids help most people with hearing loss, they do have limitations. A hearing aid is designed to restore sounds that a damaged ear can no longer distinguish properly. But even the most finely tuned sound from a hearing aid must pass through the same damaged ear, so the result is often less than perfect. Also, it takes time to get used to wearing a hearing aid—usually at least four to six weeks. Most people will need to return for adjustments more than once.

An audiologist can help you sort through all these options. But because hearing aids don't restore your hearing to normal, it is important to define how the hearing loss affects your life and therefore what your needs are. This information enables a professional to make the most appropriate recommendation for you. For instance, a business person who takes clients out to dinner on a regular basis may prefer a hearing aid with the most sophisticated degree of noise control, since there is an increased need to hear in a noisy environment. If your career requires you to conduct business primarily on a cellphone, you might prefer a hearing aid that streams sound from a phone. While many types offer this type of streaming, some may perform that particular function better than others. Your audiologist

SPECIAL SECTION | Selecting a hearing aid

will help you select the most appropriate one. Studies have shown that the most important factor in hearing aid success is a person's motivation and expectation.

Where to buy?

Each year, people buy hearing aids that don't help them hear better. One reason is that frauds and scams involving hearing aids are common. Some disreputable dispensers sell hearing aids to people who don't need them. Others talk people into buying the most expensive hearing aids and neglect to mention less costly options. Still others fit their clients poorly, so that the devices are uncomfortable or don't work well. For years, hearing aid dispensers have advertised to consumers in magazines and on TV, and some have even canvassed neighborhoods trying to sell hearing aids door to door.

The potential for fraud is now greater than ever because of the Internet. The Web may be a good source of information about dispensers. But do a search for the term "hearing aids" and you'll find hundreds of websites selling them, some of which will sell you a device sight unseen. You should steer clear of purchasing a hearing aid over the Internet or through a magazine ad unless you have fully researched the company and received recommendations from sources you trust, including your doctor, an audiologist, or one of the associations listed at the end of this report (see "Resources," page 48).

Finding a reputable dispenser

It's impossible to overemphasize the importance of finding an honest and qualified hearing aid dispenser. Buying a hearing aid isn't just a matter of getting the model you want for the best price. When you buy a hearing aid, you're entering into a long-term relationship with the dispenser. This person should fit the hearing aid to your ear, program it to your needs, teach you how to operate it, and offer assistance during the early weeks and months when you're adjusting to it. The dispenser will also offer you a service contract. That means that the dispenser should be there for you when your hearing aid needs to be adjusted or repaired. You need to feel confident that this person will be in business for many years to come and has your best interests in mind.

There are two kinds of specialists who are licensed to dispense hearing aids: audiologists and hearing instrument specialists. Audiologists are health care professionals with a master's or doctoral degree who are trained to test hearing, fit hearing aids, and recognize various problems in the ear. A hearing instrument specialist may or may not have a college degree, but he or she is trained to fit hearing aids. Although they have different backgrounds, audiologists and hearing instrument specialists are both qualified to fit hearing aids. They must possess a state license to practice. Here are some sources you can use to find a reputable, licensed dispenser:

Your doctor. Ask your primary care doctor, or seek out an otolaryngologist or otologist. These medical doctors work regularly with audiologists, sometimes in the same medical practice.

Other people with hearing aids. Ask them for the names of practitioners they've used and whether they're satisfied.

Professional organizations. The International Hearing Society, the organization of hearing instrument specialists, can refer you to a board-certified specialist in your area. The American Speech-Language-Hearing Association, a national professional

> ### ▶ Will a hearing aid help?
>
> If you think you need a hearing aid, you probably do, especially if you find that your struggles to hear are interfering in any way with your day-to-day life. That may seem obvious, yet doctors, audiologists, and patients frequently rely on hearing tests to decide whether a hearing aid will be useful. Interestingly, one of the most important predictors of hearing aid success is a person's motivation. If you think your hearing problem is a handicap, you are more likely to notice improvements with a hearing aid than someone who doesn't think his or her hearing problem is a handicap, regardless of test results.

and credentialing association for audiologists, and the American Academy of Audiology, a national professional association, can refer you to an audiologist in your area. (For information on all three groups, see "Resources," page 48.)

Signing a contract

Before you buy a hearing aid, it's a good idea to meet with more than one qualified hearing aid dispenser so that you can compare prices and service contracts. Evaluate the service contracts carefully. A contract should allow you to get a partial refund if the hearing aid you buy doesn't work out for you after about a month. If you want to return the hearing aid during or at the end of your defined trial period, you should receive a full refund for the hearing aid itself, but it's fair for the audiologist or other dispenser to be paid for the time spent fitting and adjusting it. If the contract requires you to pay in full for the hearing aid even if it proves unhelpful to you, consider going elsewhere.

Choosing a style

When you first talk with your audiologist about hearing aid options, you'll have a lot of technical terms thrown at you. The following discussion will familiarize you with the terms for hearing aid styles. Remember, you can choose different circuitry for various styles (see "Choosing circuitry," page 31). Still, as a general rule,

Wireless interfaces

A variety of wireless interfaces are available. These pick up signals from compatible devices, such as TVs, cellphones, microphones, and other audio devices, and deliver the sound directly to your hearing aids. The interfaces shown here come from Phonak, but all of the major hearing aid manufacturers have similar products that are compatible with their own brands of hearing aids.

TV connector

This device is designed to connect with your television so that you can stream your favorite TV shows directly to your compatible hearing aids. Your audiologist will help you select the best device to meet your needs.

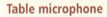

Table microphone

This two-part device is designed for meetings. You place the round component in the center of the table. It is equipped with a number of microphones pointing in different directions. The handheld control enables you to point at the person speaking, activating the microphone that is best positioned to pick up the speaker's voice.

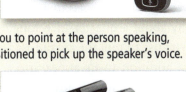

Handheld microphone

This wireless microphone works via FM signal and is recommended for people whose hearing is so impaired that any interference makes hearing difficult. You can hold it in your hand, place it on a table, wear it around your neck, or tuck it into a suit jacket pocket. You can also accept incoming calls on your cellphone using the microphone and have the sound streamed directly into your hearing aids.

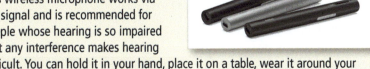

Photos courtesy of Phonak.

the smaller and less conspicuous the hearing aid, the fewer options you have for features, such as wireless capability or rechargeable batteries (a newer feature on certain behind-the-ear models). Also keep in mind that price is driven by technology rather than by style, with the exception of the completely-in-the-canal (CIC) hearing aid (discussed below) and the new

invisible models, which are consistently the most expensive in their technology bracket. Table 2, page 26, gives a quick comparison of the various models.

Over all, hearing aids have become more powerful and perform better while contained in smaller packages than ever before. All the models listed here (starting with the three smallest) have

SPECIAL SECTION | Selecting a hearing aid

become sleeker than they were and are available in more colors. Newer models are more water resistant and better at controlling noise than their predecessors.

Completely-in-the-canal (CIC)

This is a very small hearing aid—about the size of a jellybean, only slimmer. As its name indicates, it fits entirely into the ear canal. Someone looking directly at your ear from the front can't see the hearing aid, although it is partially visible from the side. As with other hearing aids, you take the device out before sleeping and before showering. (It's attached to a cord, usually about a quarter-inch long, that you use to pull the aid out.)

In addition to its appearance, a CIC hearing aid has advantages over most of the larger models. Because the CIC hearing aid lies deeper in the ear, it doesn't need as much volume as other hearing aids to give you the same degree of hearing improvement. This deep fit allows the "pinna effect," by which the outer ear helps you locate where a sound is coming from, to remain intact. CIC hearing aids can be very comfortable to wear when talking on the telephone, as the aid doesn't bump up against the receiver.

That said, CIC hearing aids have limitations. They are helpful only for mild or moderate hearing loss, not for severe hearing loss. And they're a poor choice for

Continued on page 28

Table 2: Pros and cons of various hearing aid styles

	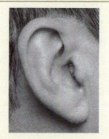**COMPLETELY-IN-THE-CANAL (CIC)**	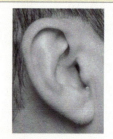**INVISIBLE-IN-THE-CANAL (IIC)**	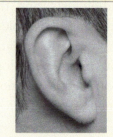**LYRIC EXTENDED-WEAR**
	The size of a jellybean, custom-made to fit deeper inside the ear canal than the more traditional styles.	Even smaller than the CIC and custom-made to fit even deeper, past the second bend of the ear canal.	Also smaller than the CIC, and placed deeper than the IIC, just 4 millimeters from the eardrum. These can be worn continuously for up to four months and are replaced by an audiologist. They are sold on a yearly subscription basis.
ADVANTAGES	Inconspicuous. Fits comfortably into most ear canal shapes and sizes. Most widely used and accepted of the custom-style hearing aids. Comfortable to use when speaking on the phone. Lasts three to five years.	Completely invisible from outside the ear. Doesn't interfere with the ear's natural ability to funnel sound (the pinna effect).	Completely invisible from outside the ear. Can be worn while sleeping, showering, and exercising. Doesn't interfere with the ear's natural ability to funnel sound (the pinna effect). The closer proximity to the eardrum helps reduce feedback.
DISADVANTAGES	Amplification is less than with larger models. Subject to wax buildup, requiring frequent cleaning or repair. Can be hard to get in and out of the ear. Difficult to manage for people with poor dexterity. No directional microphone.	Size limits features available on other hearing aids that enable hearing in all situations; amplification less than with larger models. Can be difficult to get in and out of the ear. Difficult to manage for people with poor dexterity.	Size limits features. Some ear canals too narrow or short for the device. Requires repeat visits to the audiologist for replacement when battery dies. Payment is annual for multiple hearing aids rather than once for a single device.
COST	Generally more expensive	More expensive	Most expensive option
WHO SHOULD CONSIDER IT?	People with mild to moderate hearing loss	People with mild to moderate hearing loss who do not want to be seen wearing hearing aids	People with mild to moderate hearing loss who do not want to be seen wearing hearing aids
WIRELESS CAPABILITY	No	No	No

Photos courtesy of Phonak.

Selecting a hearing aid | **SPECIAL SECTION**

IN-THE-CANAL (ITC)	IN-THE-EAR (ITE)	BEHIND-THE-EAR (BTE)	RECEIVER-IN-THE-CANAL (RIC) BTE	RECHARGEABLE BTE
Custom-made to fit into the opening of the ear canal. Only partially visible in the outer cavity of the ear.	A hollow, acrylic shell containing the circuitry is created from an impression of your ear. It fits in the outer cavity of the ear.	A case containing the receiver, microphone, and other circuitry is worn behind the ear. A narrow tube carries sound from the case to an earmold custom-made to fit in the opening of the ear.	A receiver sits inside an earbud worn in the ear canal, separating it from the microphone and amplifier, which are in a case behind the ear. A wire insulated in a thin tube connects the receiver to the BTE case.	Similar to a standard BTE or RIC BTE, except that it includes a rechargeable battery.
Provides more amplification than CIC models. Can accommodate a directional microphone system. Most models have room for a program button and/or volume control. Lasts three to five years.	Provides more amplification than some other models. Controls are easy to use. Good option for people with poor dexterity. Can accommodate a directional microphone system. Most models have room for a program button and/or volume control. Lasts three to five years.	Reliable, durable, easy to adjust the volume, easy to clean and repair. Helps the widest range of hearing loss, from mild to profound. Produces less feedback than other models. Can accommodate a directional microphone system. Long lasting.	The separation of the microphone and receiver diminishes feedback. Accommodates a wide range of hearing loss, from mild to severe. Uses directional microphones. The earmold can be close-fitted or have an open fit depending on the degree of the hearing loss. Some new models are rechargeable.	Accommodates a wide range of hearing loss, from mild to severe. Uses directional microphones. The earmold can be open or closed to accommodate varying degrees of hearing loss. Circuitry is protected from moisture in most models. Cosmetically pleasing.
Volume controls are smaller and harder to use than on larger models. Amplification is less than with larger models. Subject to wax buildup. Fitting can be difficult for people with very small ear canals.	Bulky and more visible than smaller models. Can feel hot in the ear during warm weather.	More conspicuous than other styles; feels heavier on top of the ear. May be more subject to wind noise. Harder to use with a phone.	Available in an array of sizes, but smaller ones can be difficult to manipulate. Changing the battery can be difficult for people with poor dexterity. Harder to use with a phone.	If you don't charge the hearing aids, they will not work, and charging may take hours. (Some models let you switch to a conventional battery in the meantime.) Harder to use with a phone.
Moderately expensive	Moderately expensive	Moderately expensive	Moderately expensive	Moderately expensive
People with mild to moderate hearing loss	People with mild to moderately severe hearing loss (up to 75 dB)	Adults with mild to profound hearing loss; good choice for children because of its durability and adaptability	People with mild to severe hearing loss; people concerned about the appearance of the hearing aid	People with mild to severe hearing loss; people with poor dexterity or low vision; people who work or play around water or in areas of high humidity
Some models	Most models	Most models	Most models	Most models

SPECIAL SECTION | Selecting a hearing aid

Continued from page 26

people who have a lot of earwax or fluid draining from their ears, since earwax and fluid can damage the hearing aid. In addition, people with unusually small, twisted, or angular ear canals have great difficulty wearing this style, because it is extremely difficult to maneuver the device in and out of the canal.

CIC hearing aids are too small to have certain features that add convenience and quality, particularly directional microphones (which reduce sounds in the periphery when you are in a noisy environment) and volume controls. Some are too small to have program switches. The volume level and program are preset by the hearing aid dispenser to accommodate your type of hearing loss and the range of "listening environments" that you experience regularly—for instance, a quiet evening at home one day, a noisy theater the next, and many phone conversations. If the volume setting is too loud or too soft for you, you can take it back to your hearing aid dispenser to have it adjusted. It's not unusual for people to go back several times before getting the volume and other settings just right. With some CIC models, you can get a remote control to lower the volume when you're in a very noisy place and raise the volume when you're straining to hear someone with a very soft voice.

A final drawback is the cost. CIC hearing aids tend to be among the most expensive styles, ranging from about $1,700 to $3,500 apiece depending on the level of technology of the hearing aid. More importantly, they have the shortest battery life—expect to replace the battery every three to five days. (A few companies offer rechargeable hearing aid options, but not in a CIC model.)

There are currently no wireless features with CIC hearing aids because of their small size. Wireless technology is bulky, so in general, these features are more widely available in larger hearing aids. However, the first wireless model is scheduled for release in late 2019.

Invisible-in-the-canal (IIC)

Advances in digital technology have led to development of hearing aids that are even smaller than the CIC aids. An IIC hearing aid is placed even deeper into the ear canal, past the second bend. It is completely invisible from any view of the ear, making it a nice option for people with mild or moderate hearing loss who aren't happy with more visible choices. It is essentially a smaller version of the CIC type, with fewer features. As with CIC models, the deep placement of the IIC aid preserves the natural function of the ear, perhaps even more so, enabling the pinna effect.

However, all of the disadvantages associated with CIC hearing aids described above also apply to the IIC type, including the lack of wireless capability. It is very difficult to manipulate and is removed from the ear with a longer wire than used for the CIC models, since it is placed deeper in the ear canal. Also, because of its deeper placement, there are even more restrictions on fitting, so a person must have just the right shape and size of ear canal to wear it. Since cost is driven by technology and size, these tend to be among the most expensive hearing aids, with prices ranging from $2,500 to $3,700 for a single aid.

Lyric extended-wear

The Lyric extended-wear hearing aid is also smaller than CIC models and is placed even deeper than IIC models, just 4 millimeters from the eardrum. What makes this hearing aid unique is that, unlike all others, it is disposable and can be worn while sleeping, showering, and exercising. Lyric hearing aids are worn 24 hours a day, seven days a week, and have a battery life of up to four months, at which time they are replaced by an audiologist. They are completely invisible to anyone looking at you; they remove all feeling of bulk from the ear canal for the wearer; and they offer an even more enhanced pinna effect. According to the manufacturer, Phonak Hearing Systems, the closer proximity to the eardrum also minimizes feedback (the noise that results when amplified sound is picked up again by a microphone).

The Lyric has most of the same

limitations in features and fit as the CIC and IIC hearing aids. However, because you don't have to take them out every night, you don't have to worry about the difficulty of removing and reinserting them. Most settings are preprogrammed by the hearing aid dispenser, although you can adjust certain settings along with the volume, and you can turn them on and off.

The Lyric is not for everyone, however. Because these hearing aids are placed deeper in the ear canal, the biggest drawback for many people is that the shape or size of their ear canal doesn't allow for a good fit. The Lyric can also pose problems for people who are prone to earwax impaction or those, such as people with diabetes, who are at greater risk of infection.

These hearing aids are the most expensive, as they are sold on a subscription basis. An annual subscription costs $3,400 (or $1,700 if you use only one hearing aid), covering the cost of the three new pairs of hearing aids (or individual aids) that you will need over the year.

In-the-canal (ITC)

If you can't wear a CIC hearing aid (or the other, smaller models), you might be a good candidate for an in-the-canal hearing aid, which is the next size up. This model fits just into the opening of the ear canal, so it's an option for people whose ear canals are the right size but the wrong shape for a CIC

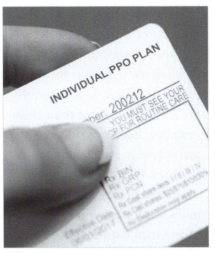

Hearing aids are expensive, and they are not covered by most insurance plans, including Medicare Part B, though some Medicare Advantage plans will give partial payment.

hearing aid. In addition, people who are too hard of hearing for a CIC model might be helped by an ITC hearing aid because it has stronger amplification. It's usually good enough to help people with moderate hearing loss. However, as with the CIC models, people who have a lot of earwax or fluid draining from their ears shouldn't use ITC hearing aids.

Unlike CIC hearing aids, ITC models are large enough to have volume controls on the hearing aids themselves, and most can also accommodate a program button and directional microphones. Some of the larger ITC hearing aids have wireless features. Ask the dispenser which controls are standard on the model you are considering. Volume and directional controls are advantages for people who want to be able to adjust the volume and to program settings as needed. However, when the volume is increased to its maximum, or when the tiny hearing aid is fitted with options to boost power, you may get feedback. Prices of ITC hearing aids range from about $1,400 to $3,500 per aid.

In-the-ear (ITE)

The next size up, the in-the-ear model, fits just outside the ear canal and fills the visible portion of the ear called the auricle (see Figure 1, page 2). Because it's been around since the early 1970s, it may seem a bit old-fashioned, particularly to people who want a hearing aid that's less noticeable. But it remains on the market because it has certain advantages over the newer, smaller hearing aids.

An ITE hearing aid can help people with hearing loss ranging from mild to severe. Compared with ITC hearing aids, the aid is larger and easier to manipulate, which is a plus for people with arthritis or others who find themselves all thumbs with small gadgets. Furthermore, this model can house a directional microphone system to help someone with mild to severe hearing loss whose difficulty includes trouble hearing speech in a noisy environment like a restaurant. ITE hearing aids can also house volume control and wireless features.

The most common complaint about this type of hearing aid is its bulky size. Another issue is that it can make the ear feel uncom-

SPECIAL SECTION | Selecting a hearing aid

fortably hot in warm weather, although this is a problem to some degree even with the smaller hearing aids. This may not be an issue at all if you don't spend much time outdoors in the heat. ITE hearing aids range from about $1,400 to $3,500 for one aid.

Behind-the-ear (BTE)

This is the oldest and largest style of hearing aid in general use, and it's the only one that doesn't contain all of its circuitry in the earmold. However, today's models are slimmer and more attractive than in the past. The electronic components are housed in a plastic case that hooks behind the ear. A fairly thin tube carries amplified sound from the circuitry to an earmold that fills the space outside the ear canal.

Despite its age, the standard BTE hearing aid is still in high demand. One reason for its enduring popularity is that it is the most powerful hearing aid on the market. While it's appropriate for all types of hearing loss, it's the only option for people with severe to profound hearing loss. This style, too, can accommodate directional microphones and wireless capability. It's also highly durable, which makes it the hearing aid of choice for children. In addition, its larger size makes it easy to change the battery, adjust the volume, turn the hearing aid on and off, and clean it—all advantages for people with limited dexterity.

Yet another explanation for the popularity of the standard BTE is that it produces minimal feedback, even when the volume is turned up high. That's because the components are farther apart than those in smaller hearing aids. Newer models provide even better control of feedback than previous BTEs.

Finally, many hearing aid manufacturers are now producing their own earmolds (the piece of the BTE that fits into the ear canal rather than sitting behind the ear; see Figure 5, page 21) instead of outsourcing this process (see "Making the earmold or shell," page 35). This allows for an acoustically optimized fit that takes into account the shape and size of a person's ear, the degree of hearing loss, and the configuration of the hearing loss as seen on the audiogram.

BTE hearing aids range in price from $1,400 to $3,500 each.

Rechargeable BTEs. Another desirable feature of newer BTEs is that some are rechargeable. This option is particularly beneficial for people who have dexterity concerns or difficulty inserting a tiny disposable battery into a hearing aid. While these BTEs are a bit bigger than others, they are more streamlined than those of the past. There are two types of rechargeable hearing aids.

With one type, the battery is built into the hearing aid. The batteries last three to five years, but they need to be recharged every one to two days. A benefit of this type of hearing aid is that it is more resistant to moisture, because the case does not have a compartment cover that you have to open repeatedly to change the battery. The solid case prevents humidity or sweat from getting inside, where the wiring and circuitry are housed. The downside is you have to remember to charge the aids (a full charge takes three hours), or else you won't be able to hear.

With the second type, a rechargeable battery can be removed from the hearing aid, so if you want to use a regular disposable hearing aid battery, instead of recharging, you have that option. The rechargeable battery must be in place in the aid when it is inserted into the charging station. The downside of this option is that the batteries expire after one year, and they cost $50 to $60 to replace.

Receiver-in-the-canal (RIC) BTE

Although the open-fit mini (see "Goodbye, feedback," page 31) is no longer actively marketed, it was a game changer that led to the development of another mini BTE model, commonly known as

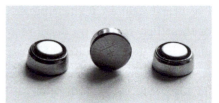

Changing the batteries in hearing aids can be an issue for people who have problems with manual dexterity. Rechargeable BTEs can help with that.

Goodbye, feedback

At one time, hearing aids needed to completely block the ear canal in order to prevent the amplified sound from leaking out of the earpiece and being picked up by the hearing aid's microphone, causing feedback. The tight fit of traditional hearing aids prevented much of this sound leakage, but it also produced a less natural sound.

With the development of feedback cancellation circuits, hearing aids with a more open fit became a possibility. The so-called open-fit mini was a game changer, offering a combination of natural and amplified sounds. You wore a small case containing the receiver, microphone, and other circuitry behind the ear, while a thin tube carried the sound from the case to a small earbud, leaving most of the ear canal open.

Today, more advanced receiver-in-the-canal hearing aids have even better feedback control, and the fitting can be either open or closed, so the open-fit mini is no longer marketed. However, some of the new over-the-counter hearing aids (see "Coming soon: Over-the-counter hearing aids," page 37) may draw on open-fit technology.

---

an RIC or RITE (receiver-in-the-ear) hearing aid. The RIC is very similar to the open-fit mini, the biggest difference being that the receiver (that is, the loudspeaker that directs amplified sound into the ear) is placed inside the ear canal instead of behind it. A thin wire insulated in a thin tube that is almost impossible to see connects the receiver to the BTE case behind the ear. The receiver is housed inside an earmold or insert that can be vented or unvented. (A vent is a hole that allows a certain amount of natural sound to enter the ear canal.)

The main advantage of an RIC is that it can accommodate people with severe hearing loss as well as those with mild hearing loss. In addition, the microphone and receiver—which are housed together in other BTE types—sit far apart from each other, allowing the wearer to enjoy a truer, richer sound, with less feedback than some other hearing aids.

The popularity of the RIC has led manufacturers to produce some with unique shapes and fashionable colors and textures to accommodate personal style. It also comes in a wide variety of sizes.

Although it sounds like the perfect hearing aid, as it's one of the least noticeable and has the power to accommodate severe hearing loss, the RIC does have some drawbacks. Its smaller size makes it difficult to manipulate. For those with dexterity concerns, changing the battery can be hard. Another disadvantage is that the location of the microphone behind the ear makes it harder to use with a phone. RICs range from $1,400 to $3,500 each. Some models have wireless capability.

Rechargeable RICs. A brand new feature of some RICs is that they are rechargeable. Two basic versions exist (see "Rechargeable BTEs," page 30).

Choosing circuitry

The quality of the sound you get from your hearing aid depends on the circuitry you choose. Digital hearing aid circuitry was introduced in 1996, and it has since rendered analog technology obsolete, as even the most basic entry-level digital hearing aids rivaled analog hearing aids in price and outperformed them in features.

The benefit of digital technology is that a digital device can perform many complicated functions at great speed. Digital hearing aids automatically separate incoming sound into different frequency regions. Think of these as buckets. The hearing aid can then automatically prioritize and amplify or diminish sound from each bucket selectively, depending on the wearer's hearing loss profile. There are several tiers of digital hearing aids available. Premium-level technology—the most expensive—offers the most buckets to manage sounds more precisely. It also offers the most features, like directional microphones, noise cancellation systems, and feedback management. Advanced-level circuitry offers many of the same features, but over all has less flexibility

SPECIAL SECTION | Selecting a hearing aid

to deal with complex listening situations. Entry-level digital circuits naturally have the fewest features.

All hearing aids are equipped with three basic parts: a microphone to collect sounds, a circuit to amplify sounds, and a receiver that sends the sounds into your ear. Beyond that, hearing aids have several optional features.

Directional microphones. Two or more microphones are placed and matched in such a way as to improve the signal-to-noise ratio—that is, the measure of what you want to hear (the signal) relative to what you don't want to hear (the noise). A +6 dB signal-to-noise ratio, meaning that the signal is 6 dB louder than the noise, is the level often found to make a noticeable improvement in understanding speech in a noisy environment. A directional microphone system is the best way to achieve this +6 dB level. Directional microphones are available in most hearing aids except for CIC, IIC, and extended-wear styles. Some models turn on the directional microphone program automatically, while others require the wearer to turn it on by pushing on the hearing aid.

Telecoil. A telecoil, or t-coil, is a small copper coil that converts acoustic energy from a targeted source, bridging the space between a hearing aid and that source. It is located inside the hearing aid, and you can turn it on and off as necessary by pressing a button on the aid. (Because the t-coil is relatively large, it's only found on the larger hearing aid models—BTEs, RICs, most ITEs, and some ITCs.) Originally t-coils were used primarily to boost the signals from a telephone handset or cellphone. But with the explosion of new wireless technologies, uses for t-coils have expanded. They can now be used in conjunction with assistive listening devices (see "The digital revolution," page 20), and they enable you to hear in public venues via a hearing loop—a wire that encircles a room and connects directly to its sound system. The loop transmits the sound electromagnetically, and the electromagnetic signal is picked up by the t-coil in the hearing aid. The use of looping is rapidly expanding in public places, such as theatres, train stations,

Figure 6: T-coil sign

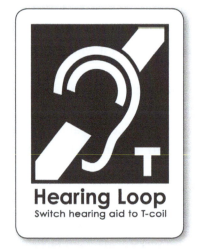

This symbol indicates that a public venue is looped—that is, equipped with technology that transmits signals from the room's sound system directly to telecoil-enabled hearing aids.

airports, and places of worship. In public places that are looped, you will see a sign for the telecoil (see Figure 6, below).

Landline telephone features. The t-coil converts acoustic energy from the phone to electric energy, enabling the hearing aid to communicate with a landline telephone without the feedback that can occur when a telephone receiver is held very near a hearing aid. To turn it on, you push a button on the hearing aid—or with some models, the t-coil switches on automatically when the telephone receiver is placed at the ear.

Cellphone features. Hearing aids and cellphones are not easily compatible—especially if you're using a t-coil. That's because the transmitter and the antenna of a cellphone emit radiofrequencies (RF) that create an audible sound when a hearing aid is placed near the phone. However, some cellphones are more compatible with hearing aids than others because their RF emissions are low. Regulations from the Federal Communications Commission make it easier to find these phones. According to these regulations, cellphones must display a rating from 1 to 4 for reduced RF interference. This rating must be visible on the packaging of all hearing aid–compatible cellphones. The higher the rating, the clearer the sound. So, when shopping for a cellphone, look for a microphone (M) rating of M3 or M4 if your hearing aid does not have a t-coil. This means the cellphone will work with the hearing aid in microphone mode. If your hearing aid has a t-coil, look for a rating of T3 or T4.

All nationwide cellphone retailers must meet a minimum of an M3 rating for at least 50% or eight of their handheld cellphones, whichever is less, in addition to a T3 rating for one-third or seven of their handset models.

When shopping for a cellphone, look for the highest combination of M and T ratings on the cellphone packaging. The higher the result, the better the connection with less noise. Although these ratings are extremely useful, be sure to try several cellphone models with your hearing aid before you buy, and listen to the difference yourself.

Automatic gain control (AGC). This is a volume control feature found in most modern hearing aids. The goal of amplification is to make soft sounds audible, moderate sounds comfortable and clear, and loud sounds tolerable. AGC systems make these adjustments automatically, as opposed to requiring the user to manually adjust the volume.

Feedback management. These systems are used to reduce or eliminate feedback. In the past, eliminating feedback usually meant reducing the gain (power) of the hearing aid. This reduced the benefit of the hearing aid as well. Newer feedback management systems are able to detect the whistling sound and create an identical signal in the opposite phase, thereby canceling the feedback. This happens very quickly, without any action on the part of the wearer.

Noise cancellation systems. These reduce steady-state noise. Steady-state noises are those that follow a repeatable and predictable pattern, like air vents and fans. Noise cancellation algorithms are able to detect these steady-state noise patterns and significantly reduce them. This means the wearer is less bothered by routine environmental sounds. Wind noise, a common problem with older-model hearing aids, is addressed by more advanced circuits, which are able to reduce the static sound that occurs when wind passes over the microphone of a hearing aid.

Multiple programs. These are available in most hearing aids. The frequency response that offers the best amplification varies based on the environment. For example, the optimum settings for quiet environments are different from the optimum settings for noisy environments, and different still for specific situations like music, lectures, or theater performances. With multiple programs, a user can access various settings by pushing a button on the hearing aid or using a remote control. However, the need for pushing buttons is shifting with technology, as it becomes more common for hearing aids to have advanced circuits that automatically select the appropriate program based on the surroundings.

One hearing aid or two?

If you're like most people with hearing loss, you'll probably find that it takes time to accept the idea that you need a hearing aid, and you may be unhappy when your audiologist recommends that you get not one, but two. Chances are that your first question will be, "Is it normal to get two hearing aids?" And then, "Do I really need two?"

If you have hearing loss in only one ear and normal or nearly normal hearing in the other, then one hearing aid is all you need. But most people have hearing loss in both ears, especially if the loss is age-related. (You may have one ear that's better than the other, but chances are both will be in the same ballpark.) In that case, research and experience suggest that you'll ultimately be more satisfied with two hearing aids.

When you have two hearing aids, you can take better advantage of the way the brain processes sound through what's known as binaural hearing. With normal hearing, sound signals from both ears are comparable in strength. The brain can pick out the important signals, like voices, when they're louder than the background noise. But if you're wearing just one hearing aid and someone talks into your unaided ear in a noisy room, the voice may sound softer than the background noise. As a result, it's harder for your brain to give it preferential status.

It may also be harder for the brain to identify the location of particular sounds if you're wearing a single hearing aid. The brain normally does this by comparing the qualities of the sound signals that come through each ear—their relative loudness, their frequencies, and the time it takes them to travel through the ears. But the brain can't locate a sound as well if sound signals are always louder through one ear.

Wearing wireless hearing aids in both ears enhances the binaural hearing process because the hearing aids communicate with each other and transfer data back and forth, rather than working independently to process sound. This means they are able to maintain localization cues better than hearing aids working independently of each other.

Some hearing experts think that wearing two hearing aids may even help conserve hearing in the weaker ear by keeping the auditory nerve stimulated with adequately amplified sound. There's no proof that the auditory nerves actually deteriorate from inadequate stimulation, but research shows that other parts of the nervous system—most notably the brain—do suffer from lack of use.

One undisputed advantage of wearing two hearing aids is that you can set them at a lower volume than if you wear just one. That's because soft tones sound louder when the brain is receiving signals from two ears rather than one. And lower volume means less feedback. If your audiologist recommends two hearing aids and you're not sure that you want or need two, ask if you can use two on a trial basis. Under this arrangement, you would be fitted with two hearing aids and then, over a period of several weeks, you would decide whether you hear better with two. If not, you should be able to return one of them. Keep in mind that if you want to take advantage of wireless features, both hearing aids must be wireless.

Fitting a hearing aid

Once you select the style and circuitry of your hearing aid, the dispenser will need to fit the hearing

---

Hearing loss and the law

People with hearing loss are protected from discrimination and are entitled to certain services under the federal Americans with Disabilities Act. The act prohibits employers from discriminating against job applicants and employees who are hard of hearing. And it requires businesses, government agencies, medical establishments, and service providers to remove barriers to people with hearing impairments.

In essence, institutions must enable people who are hard of hearing to communicate to the same degree as people with normal hearing. Telephone companies must provide telecommunications devices for the deaf, or TDDs, upon request at no extra charge. These devices allow deaf users to send and receive typed messages over the telephone. Hotels and other public accommodations are required to provide TDDs to guests, as are shopping malls, stadiums, hospital waiting rooms, airports, and any other building with more than four pay phones. Cellular phone providers must have cellphone models that are compatible with hearing aids and must allow consumers to test them before buying them (see "Cellphone features," page 32).

The law requires businesses, government facilities, and federally funded hospitals to provide assistance in communicating, but the burden is on you to say what type of assistance you need. It can be an interpreter to help you understand medical information or something as simple as a pencil and paper to write down questions. If you stay overnight in a hospital that receives federal funds, the hospital must provide a TDD as well as television captioning.

The government has two toll-free telephone numbers you can call to file discrimination complaints. For employer complaints, call the U.S. Equal Employment Opportunity Commission at 800-669-4000 (voice) or 800-669-6820 (TDD). If you have been denied a service, call the Department of Justice's Americans with Disabilities Act information line at 800-514-0301 (voice) or 800-514-0383 (TDD).

Selecting a hearing aid | **SPECIAL SECTION**

aid. Fitting is a multistep process that usually includes not only creating an earmold or shell that fits your ear, but also programming or adjusting the hearing aid so that it's helpful for your particular kind of hearing loss and lifestyle. Fitting also involves teaching you how to use the aid.

Making the earmold or shell. First, the dispenser puts a soft, squishy material in and around your ear to make an impression for the mold. For most hearing aid styles, an impression is made of your ear canal and outer ear. It takes five to 10 minutes for the material to harden. Then the dispenser sends the impression to the hearing aid manufacturer to make a custom earmold or shell. The manufacturer will send the finished hearing aid to your dispenser roughly one to three weeks later.

Assessing or adjusting the fit. When the hearing aid arrives, the dispenser will put it in your ear to see how well it fits. It should be secure enough not to slip or fall out when you move your head. If the hearing aid moves around, it will likely create feedback. Although the hearing aid will probably feel strange at first simply because you've never worn one before, it shouldn't be uncomfortable. If it is, tell your dispenser. If the dispenser can't make the hearing aid feel comfortable, you'll need to have a new ear impression made.

Programming the hearing aid. Next, the dispenser will program your hearing aid to meet your particular needs by hooking it up to a computer loaded with software that incorporates your audiogram results and your hearing aid settings.

Learning to use the device. When the earmold or shell fits properly and the aid is programmed properly, the dispenser will teach you how to use the hearing aid. This includes learning how to put it in and take it out, use it with your telephone, and, if applicable, adjust the volume and change the programs. You'll also learn the essentials of maintaining your hearing aid, like how and when to clean it, how to change the battery, and how to tell if the battery is low.

Going for a test drive. After the programming is complete, you'll insert your new hearing aid (or aids) for a test run. Don't expect to hear as well as you did when your hearing was normal. Sounds heard through a hearing aid are like recorded music: they can come close to the real thing, but they're not quite as clear or as natural. However, sounds shouldn't be so unnatural that they're bothersome. If they are—if voices sound tinny, for example—the hearing aid dispenser can improve the sound quality by adjusting various amplification parameters. The degree

---

Personal sound amplification products (PSAPs)

Personal sound amplification products (PSAPs) have gotten a lot of attention in recent years. These are more affordable devices that can benefit people with mild hearing loss, but they are not hearing aids and therefore they are not regulated by the FDA as medical devices for the hearing impaired. Some, like the Bose Hearphones, have a semicircular piece you wear around your neck; this neckpiece connects to wires that lead into earphones. Like other Bose products, they have excellent sound reproduction, especially for music—and they offer noise cancellation to filter out distracting sounds—but they don't function like hearing aids.

PSAPs simply amplify sound. They do not address other hearing issues such as distortion. They are sold without a prescription (primarily online) and are self-fitted, coming in generic sizes like small, medium, and large rather than being molded to fit your ear canal. You can program them yourself using a smartphone or computer app. Most cost somewhere between $250 and $350 apiece, although some can cost up to $1,000 or more.

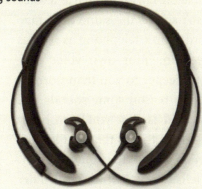

PSAPs like the Bose Hearphones amplify sounds but do not have other features.

---

www.health.harvard.edu

Coping with Hearing Loss 35

of fine-tuning that can be done depends on which circuitry you have. Don't be shy about asking your dispenser to keep fine-tuning your hearing aid until you're satisfied. That's part of what you're paying for. But be realistic about the sound quality that the hearing aid can provide.

Measuring the results. An important step during the fitting process is to test how well your hearing aid is working for you. Real ear testing (or probe microphone testing) measures how accurately sound is amplified by your hearing aid and how well it resonates in the ear. The dispenser will place a tiny microphone inside your ear canal and hook it up to a computer. Then he or she will adjust the programming until the amplification is at its best. This test is especially helpful for young children, who can't always reliably report the sounds and words they hear.

Another test, called functional gain testing, involves wearing your hearing aid while listening to and then repeating sounds and words spoken to you—sometimes with a lot of background noise and other times with very little. How accurately you pick up the sounds and repeat the words indicates how well the hearing aid is working for you. The dispenser will keep adjusting the controls on your hearing aid until you're able to hear as well as possible.

Not all dispensers give these tests, but they can provide important information about whether the hearing aid has been fitted and programmed properly. When interviewing dispensers, ask whether they use such objective tests, and avoid those who do not use these tests or who use them only in cases where a patient is dissatisfied.

Getting used to it

Before you walk out of the dispenser's office, be sure you are reasonably comfortable with your new hearing aid. The hearing aid shouldn't slip around or hurt. Sounds should be louder than before, but not so loud that they bother your ears. For the most part, sounds shouldn't be shrill or disturbing in other ways. But that isn't to say that everything will be perfect. Hearing aids have their limitations, especially in the beginning.

The first thing many new users notice is that sounds seem strange. Remember that even the best hearing aids are not as good as natural hearing, so sounds aren't completely normal, much as a voice doesn't sound the same on a tape recorder or a telephone as it does in person. Your own voice may sound deeper to you than normal. Another reason some sounds will seem odd is that you'll probably be hearing things that you haven't heard in a long time. One audiologist tells of a patient who called her to complain about a hissing sound. It turned out that the person was hearing the radiator.

You may also be more aware than ever before of your footsteps, your car's motor, the sounds you make as you chew your food, and just about any other environmental noise. Many hearing aids can be adjusted to lower the volume of unwanted noise, but more importantly, with time, your brain will get better at tuning it out. The

> **The people who keep their hearing aids in for the longest time each day during the first few weeks adjust the fastest.**

more you wear your hearing aids, the more easily your brain will adjust to the changes.

Although background sounds will seem louder than before, you may find that the hearing aid doesn't do one of the things you'd most hoped that it would: enable you to understand every word in a conversation. Of course, you should be able to understand more words with the hearing aid than without—if you can't, the hearing aid may need some fine-tuning. But even with a hearing aid, you won't catch everything. The important thing to realize is that hearing every word isn't necessary. The goal is for you to follow conversation easily in various environments. You should continue to rely on the visual cues that you've been using all along to understand words, like lip movements, facial expressions, and hand gestures.

Getting used to a hearing aid takes time, usually at least four to six weeks, but it may take as long as several months until your ability to understand speech has peaked. If you don't notice a marked improvement by the end of the first month, there's a strong chance that the hearing aid isn't right for you. In most states, dispensers are required by law to give you a month-long trial period, which allows you to return a new hearing aid if you're not satisfied. If you return the hearing aid, you may be asked to pay a fee. If you're not sure whether you want to return it after a month, relay your concerns to your dispenser and ask if you can extend the trial period. It is important to see your dispenser regularly during the trial period to review your progress with the hearing aid.

The amount of time it takes to adjust to a new hearing aid depends on many things. The more severe your hearing loss—and the longer you waited before getting a hearing aid—the longer it will likely take you to adjust. But, as stated earlier, even more important than the severity of your hearing loss is your motivation. Audiologists say that people who really want to use their new hearing aids end up being more satisfied than those who don't.

Another factor is how much time you spend wearing your hearing aid when you first take it home. The people who keep their hearing aids in for the longest time each day during the first few weeks adjust the fastest. Don't worry about "wasting" the hearing aid battery or shutting your hearing aid off when you're home alone. Follow your dispenser's advice, but be prepared to wear your new hearing aid for several hours a day at first, and to gradually increase the time you wear it each day after that. Researchers think that wearing a hearing aid for a sustained period teaches the brain how to hear again.

Coming soon: Over-the-counter hearing aids

With the vast improvements in hearing technology, you might expect hearing aids to have grown in popularity. However, the truth is that the large majority of people with hearing loss do not seek help. Most do not get tested, and less than 20% of adults with hearing loss use a hearing aid, according to several estimates. For many people in early stages of hearing loss, social stigma discourages them from seeking treatment, but another barrier to wearing hearing aids is the cost, especially for those living in underserved communities.

As a result, the federal government passed legislation in 2017 to create a new category of hearing aid to be sold over the counter, without a prescription, to adults with mild to moderate hearing loss.

Traditionally, hearing aids have been available only through licensed professionals, and their high price tag has put them out of reach for many consumers, especially since the cost is not covered by Medicare or most insurance plans. The new hearing aids will be more affordable. In addition, the FDA announced in 2016 it would no longer enforce a requirement that individuals obtain a medical evaluation by a physician (or sign a waiver) in order to obtain these devices. At the time of this printing, the FDA had not yet finalized regulations governing over-the-counter hearing aids, and they will not be available before August 2020.

The new over-the-counter hearing aids have been dubbed "readers for the ears" in reference to the generic reading glasses you can buy in drugstores. They will provide the same basic components as a traditional hearing aid—receiver, amplifier, and distortion control—but will offer fewer features, and you will have to fit them yourself. While it is too soon to make any recommendations regarding these products, it is important to note that managing hearing loss is a complex process. If possible, it is still preferable to consult an audiologist, who can tailor custom hearing aids to your needs and preferences.

Surgery for hearing loss

Although hearing aids can help most people with hearing loss, some people may benefit instead from surgery to improve or correct their hearing. Certain kinds of hearing loss can only be treated with surgery—for example, to repair malformations in the ear, to drain fluid, to replace or reconstruct the ossicles, or to implant a device to improve hearing. Implantable devices include bone-conducting hearing aids, middle ear implants, ossicle bone–stimulating hearing aids, cochlear implants, and auditory brainstem implants. Sometimes surgery is performed to improve a person's hearing to the point that it can be helped by a hearing aid. These surgeries are typically covered by most health insurance plans. The following are the most common types of surgery for hearing problems.

Bone-conducting aids

The implantable bone-conducting hearing aid, also referred to as a bone-anchored hearing aid (BAHA) or bone-anchored hearing system (BAHS), has been on the market since the late 1990s and is intended for people who can't wear regular hearing aids, either because they have chronic ear infections or because they do not have an ear canal. It is also used on the deaf side in people with single-sided hearing loss. Unlike conventional hearing aids, which amplify sound before it passes into the ear, a bone-conducting system reroutes sound vibrations directly through your skull to your inner ear, thus bypassing the middle and outer ear entirely. Examples include the Baha (sold by Cochlear), the Ponto (Oticon), and the Sophono (Sophono).

All these systems rely on a metal screw that is surgically implanted into the skull behind the ear, where it conducts sound to the inner ear by vibrating against the mastoid bone in the skull. The screw is then connected to an external hearing aid. With the Baha and Ponto, this is done using an abutment that's attached to the screw and brought out through the skin for attachment of the hearing aid. This abutment needs to be cleaned daily to prevent a localized infection. With the Sophono, a magnet is attached to the screw and buried under the skin, with no opening through the skin. The hearing aid is then held on with the magnet. While this avoids the risk of skin infection, this device delivers somewhat less volume than the others. Therefore, the choice of system depends upon weighing the risk of infection against the need for more volume.

Middle ear implant

Another type of implant, a vibrating ossicular prosthesis, is designed for people with moderate to severe sensorineural hearing loss who have not been satisfied with hearing aids. This technology is an FDA-approved middle ear implant that improves hearing by vibrating the incus bone in the middle ear, whose oscillations are needed to initiate the chain of events that enables the brain to recognize sounds.

The implant has internal and external components. Internally, a receiver implanted behind the ear is connected to an electromagnet (about the size of a grain of rice) that's attached to the incus bone. Externally, an inch-long audio processor is held in place magnetically next to the internal receiver. The processor contains a battery, a microphone, and circuits that transmit the sound through the skin to the internal receiver. The receiver amplifies the signal and relays it to a vibrating device within the internal unit. The vibrations make the incus bone vibrate—more so than it would on its own, thus amplifying the volume of sound transmitted to the inner ear. Surgery to place the device takes about an hour and a half and is done on an outpatient basis. The device can be implanted in one or both ears, depending on your needs.

Advantages over hearing aids include comfort, better sound quality, and no feedback. In addition, you can swim with the implant, bathe with it, and sleep with it. Plus, this technology is advancing, so future models will be better, with smaller external components. Newer versions of the device allowing for connection to the stapes bone or the inner ear directly are also under development.

The main drawback is that the implant is expensive and isn't covered by Medicare, although some private insurance plans pay for it.

Cochlear implant

Cochlear implants are used for adults and children with sensorineural hearing loss in both ears that is so extreme even the best hearing aid has little or no effect. The doctor surgically implants an electrical device and later attaches external parts, including a microphone and speech processor, to restore some hearing. This surgery has helped many people who would otherwise have no hope of improving their hearing. With universal screening for newborns, increasing numbers of cochlear implants are being done on very young children.

A cochlear implant is different from a hearing aid. It bypasses the usual route of sound through the ear to the hair cells in the cochlea and then to the auditory nerve. Instead, it sends an electrical signal directly from an external antenna to the implanted receiver and then to electrodes in the inner ear, which stimulate the auditory nerve.

A cochlear implant is not an alternative to a hearing aid for people with mild to moderate hearing loss from aging or other common causes. However, as the technology continues to improve, the gap between those who can be helped by hearing aids and those who can be helped by cochlear implants is narrowing. The biggest improvement with implants is better speech and language discrimination and perception. Still, how much a person is able to hear after a cochlear implant depends on many things, including how long the person has been deaf and his or her motivation to learn how to use the implant.

The procedure carries some risks.

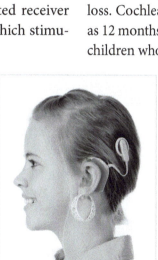

A cochlear implant is for young children or for people who have lost their hearing, not those who have always been deaf, because speech-language development of the brain is essential to success.

People with cochlear implants are more susceptible to bacterial meningitis caused by *Streptococcus pneumoniae*. Experts strongly recommend that all people with cochlear implants stay up to date with all vaccinations, particularly the pneumococcal vaccine, which protects against the most common strains of the bacteria that cause meningitis. In addition, it is important to watch for symptoms of meningitis and middle ear infection, including fever, headache, stiff neck, nausea, vomiting, irritability, discomfort looking at bright lights, sleepiness, confusion, ear pain, hearing loss, or appetite loss.

Who's a good candidate for a cochlear implant?

A cochlear implant is for young children or for people who have lost their hearing, not those who have always been deaf, because speech-language development of the brain is essential to success. Those who benefit from cochlear implants learn to associate the signal provided by an implant with sounds the brain remembers. To be a candidate, you must be in good physical health, because the procedure is a major operation done in the hospital under general anesthesia.

One of the fastest-growing age groups receiving cochlear implants is children with profound hearing loss. Cochlear implants can be given to those as young as 12 months old, as research has continued to show that children who receive cochlear implants at a younger age acquire more age-appropriate language skills than children implanted when they are older. That's because they're being exposed to sounds during a time in their development that is crucial to acquiring speech and language skills.

Children generally receive implants in both ears, since research in children has shown that this leads to better speech and language development as well as better communication skills. Adults, however, generally receive an implant in just one ear. Research is under way to determine whether a second implant improves their communication skills enough to make a second implant desirable.

The first step in finding out if a cochlear implant is right for you is to talk with an otolaryngologist or otologist who performs this surgery. The doctor will require you to have a hearing test and medical exam to determine the cause and severity of your hearing loss. The doctor may also want you to undergo psychological screening to make sure that you are mentally prepared for the rigors of rehabilitation following the surgery.

Eligibility for cochlear implants continually expands to include more people, so if your hearing loss wasn't extreme enough to qualify you for an implant several years back, you may be eligible now or in the future. In fact, newer versions of cochlear implants and new surgical techniques used in implantation sometimes enable surgeons to preserve any hearing that remains, while simulating the tones you no longer have. If you are doing well with your hearing aid, however, a cochlear implant is not recommended.

Figure 7: How a cochlear implant works

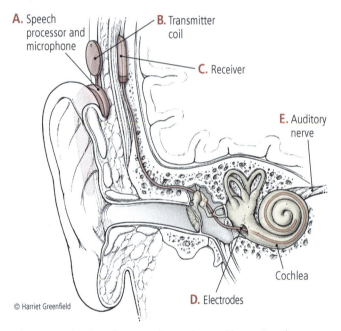

The process begins when sounds are detected by a microphone in the earpiece (A). The speech processor converts the sound waves into electrical signals and passes these along a wire to a transmitting coil that attaches behind the ear (B). The transmitter relays the signals through the skin to the implanted receiver (C), which transmits the electrical current down wires to electrodes (D) in the cochlea. These electrodes stimulate the auditory nerve (E), which sends the signal to the brain.

The surgery

The cochlear implant procedure requires general anesthesia. The surgeon first makes an incision behind the ear to reach the mastoid bone. A pocket is made behind the mastoid bone to hold the receiver unit of the implant. The mastoid cavity is opened up to make a pathway from the receiver to the cochlea. The round window (a membrane below the oval window that forms one of two entrances to the inner ear) is then opened to allow the surgeon to insert the implant electrodes into the cochlea. The opening is then sealed around the electrodes, and the implant is secured behind the mastoid. Finally the skin is stitched closed.

The term cochlear implant is a bit misleading, because not all of the components are implanted. About a month after the surgery, you will return to an audiologist to be fitted for the external components that operate the implant. You will wear a small microphone behind your ear to pick up incoming sounds. You'll also wear a speech processor. Older models, which are boxes about the size of a deck of cards, hang on a belt or are carried in a pocket, but the newer models fit right behind the ear, like a behind-the-ear hearing aid. The speech processor converts sound waves from the microphone into electrical signals, which are sent through a wire to a transmitting coil attached behind the ear. This coil then converts the signals into radio waves and sends them through the skull to the receiver, which passes them to the electrodes in the inner ear. The electrodes stimulate the auditory nerve, allowing the signal to be sent to the brain (see Figure 7, at left). Most people stay in the hospital less than 24 hours. Recovery from the surgery usually takes a few days. However, the implant is not turned on for about four weeks, to allow the soft tissue around the implant to heal properly. After that, be prepared to have rehabilitation to learn how to use the implant.

It is possible that someday fully implantable cochlear implants will be available. Efforts are already under way to develop such a system (see "In development: A fully implantable cochlear implant," page 41).

Learning to hear with a cochlear implant

Once the doctor has attached all the components, you must work with an audiologist to learn how to listen to and interpret sounds through the implant. Speech may sound mechanical and other sounds may be almost unrecognizable at first. Some people can understand words and carry on a conversation following a cochlear implant, but others have to learn how to interpret speech by using visual cues, like lip reading. During rehabilitation, you'll learn to associate the way different sounds are heard through the implant with their origin in your daily environment—the doorbell, the telephone, a car starting, and so on.

Learning to use a cochlear implant is hard work. Rehabilitation can take six months to a year for an adult and many years for a child. But the reward is that in the end, most people can understand some speech, hold conversations, and even talk on the telephone. New studies show that the longer you have the implant, the more your hearing improves, even after the first year.

Most insurance plans cover cochlear implants for people with severe sensorineural hearing loss.

Preventing infection

The Centers for Disease Control and Prevention recommends that people with cochlear implants be vaccinated against *Streptococcus pneumoniae*, the bacterium most likely to cause meningitis in people with cochlear implants. The CDC recommends pneumococcal conjugate vaccine (PCV13) for anyone who has such an implant or is scheduled for the surgery. It also recommends pneumococcal polysaccharide vaccine (PPSV23) for those ages 2 and older who have the implant or are scheduled for surgery.

Auditory brainstem implant

Some people either are born without auditory nerves or have lost them because of tumors. In these people, hearing aids or cochlear implants are not helpful, because they have no nerves connecting the ear to the brainstem, from which sound signals are relayed to the auditory cortex. For these individuals, an implant has been developed that replaces the auditory nerve. The implant replaces thousands of nerve connections with only a few, but those few are enough to restore some hearing.

As with the cochlear implant, the auditory brainstem implant includes both internal and external components. An electrode is surgically implanted in the brainstem, and a receiver is implanted in the skull bone under the skin. A microphone worn behind the ear relays incoming sounds to an external speech processor, which converts the sounds to digital signals and then sends them to a transmitter. The transmitter sends the digital sound signals to the internal components, which translate them into electrical signals to stimulate nerves in the brain.

There is a lengthy period of recuperation after surgery. About eight weeks after the surgery, you must see an audiologist to get the implant up and running. The initial work takes place in a hospital because there is a small risk that the initial electrical stimulation can affect the heart. Programming and evaluating the auditory brainstem implant takes three days, but full recovery and rehabilitation—including programming modifications and training to maximize the benefit of the implant—usually takes about a year.

Most people get one implant, but work is being done to see if two will improve the results.

Other surgeries

Several additional types of surgery are available to help correct other kinds of hearing loss.

Stapedectomy

This operation corrects otosclerosis, a common cause

> ### In development: A fully implantable cochlear implant
>
> As the technology behind cochlear implants continues to improve, the next phase of development is expected to be a totally implantable cochlear implant—although it won't be commercially available for years, even if it proves viable in testing. One cochlear implant manufacturer, Cochlear Limited, announced in October 2018 that it was launching a clinical feasibility study in Australia to evaluate performance and safety of an implanted microphone, an implanted rechargeable battery, and an implanted sound processor. With this new type of cochlear implant, a patient would have the option of using an external sound processor for better sound quality, or removing it while still maintaining hearing. Stay tuned.

Figure 8: Stapedectomy

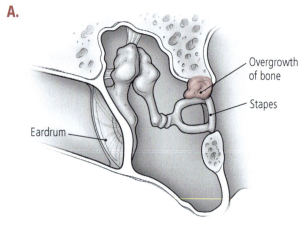

A.

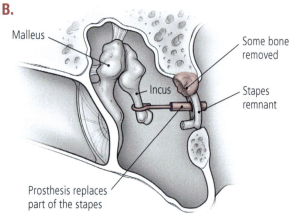

B.

An abnormal bone growth, as shown in the top drawing (A), sometimes prevents the stapes from vibrating and passing sound waves to the inner ear. To correct this condition, the surgeon removes all or part of the stapes bone and replaces it with a prosthesis (B). After surgery, sound waves pass through the eardrum to the malleus and then the incus, which is connected to the prosthesis. These vibrations cause the prosthesis to move, and the sound waves pass into the inner ear, as they should.

of conductive hearing loss characterized by abnormal growth around the stapes bone (in the middle ear) or the otic capsule (the bone surrounding the labyrinth of the inner ear). The most common location of abnormal bone growth is next to the stapes, the smallest ossicle in the middle ear. Hearing loss occurs because the abnormal bone keeps the stapes from vibrating normally and passing the sound waves from the ear canal to the inner ear. Surgery can help. Working through the ear canal, the surgeon removes all or part of the stapes and replaces it with an artificial one (see Figure 8, above). Because the stapes lies behind the eardrum, the surgeon must move the eardrum out of the way to perform the operation and then put it back.

The major risks of stapedectomy are hearing loss, dizziness, and change in taste in part of the tongue. The dizziness usually goes away, and the taste problem generally clears in a few months. However, the hearing loss can be permanent. With newer techniques and materials for reconstructing the bones, 95% of people with conductive hearing loss have their hearing restored, but in 1% of cases, the hearing loss is permanent. Some surgeons will not perform the operation unless the hearing loss is great enough to justify the risks. Discuss the risks and benefits of this operation with your doctor and, if you decide to go ahead with it, choose a surgeon who performs this operation regularly.

Tympanoplasty

If your eardrum has been ruptured by some trauma or infection and the rupture doesn't heal on its own within a few months, you may need a type of surgery called tympanoplasty to patch the hole in the eardrum. In this operation, the surgeon takes nearby tissue (fascia, cartilage, or perichondrium) and uses it to close the hole or to fashion a new eardrum.

Myringotomy

This simple outpatient procedure is performed mainly on children who have persistent fluid buildup in the middle ear, usually because of recurrent ear infections that don't respond well to antibiotics. An otolaryngologist or otologist inserts a ventilation tube into the eardrum to drain fluid from the middle ear. The tubes are left in place for six to 18 months and may be removed if they do not come out on their own.

Reconstructive surgery

This is a complex surgical procedure intended to correct structural problems of the ear, either congenital or acquired. Not all abnormalities can be corrected, but most can. Ears, ear canals, eardrums, and ossicles can usually be reconstructed to work normally. The risks, benefits, and success rates depend upon the complexity of the problem being treated. Your ear surgeon will review these with you during the discussion of treatment options.

Living well with hearing loss

Hearing loss affects more than just a person's sense of hearing. For many people, it symbolizes the loss of youthfulness or competence. Hearing loss makes people vulnerable to social isolation and depression. A hearing aid or surgery can help correct the physical problems in the ear, but it doesn't eliminate the emotional toll. If anything, a new hearing device can add to your distress at first because adjusting to one is hard, frustrating work.

That said, there are strategies you can adopt to help compensate for any remaining difficulty you have with hearing, both in the short term—as you're adapting to life with a hearing aid or surgery—and in the long term. There are also things your friends and loved ones can do to make communication easier.

While you're adjusting to hearing aids

These steps can improve your communication with others:

- Start off with one-on-one conversations—the easiest ones to understand—and gradually work up to conversations that involve three or more people.
- Realize that understanding conversations in noisy places, like restaurants and parties, will be difficult at first, but that with time and practice, your ability to hear in these settings will improve. Make a habit of watching the person who is speaking so you can pick up gestures and other visual cues to help understand what's being said. When possible, position yourself close to the person who is speaking so you can see him or her clearly.
- Don't interrupt the speaker. You may not understand the beginning of what's said, but you may pick up enough of what comes later on to get the gist of the comment.
- Don't expect to catch every word. Look for ideas instead of individual words.
- Install a telephone amplifier at home to help you hear telephone conversations.
- If using the phone is a problem, consider email or text messaging instead.
- Wear your hearing aid. The more you use it, the better your hearing will be.
- Try to keep your sense of humor. You won't understand everything that's said to you—even people with normal hearing don't. But with time and patience, you'll understand more than you did before you got your hearing aid.

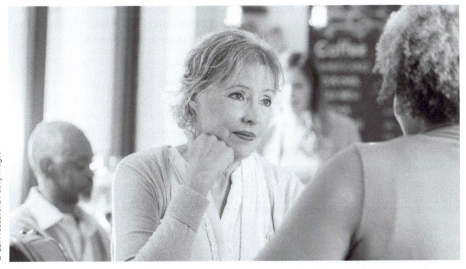

One-on-one conversations are the easiest to understand, because there are fewer distractions and you can focus on the person across from you. While you're adjusting to your hearing aids, include more of these conversations. Gradually work up to ones with larger groups of people.

Long-term strategies

Even people with completely normal hearing can be poor listeners. Listening involves thought processes, auditory memory, language skills, and

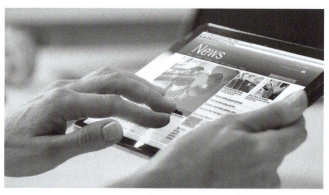

There are various ways to compensate for hearing loss in social situations. If you stay aware of current events, you'll be more likely to recognize key words, names, and concepts in converesations.

being present rather than distracted. Developing listening skills and other communications strategies as well as joining self-help groups that surround you with people who are facing the same challenges you are can be vital in getting the most out of your hearing aids. Here are some communication strategies you can practice:

- Stay aware of current events. When you know something about a topic, you can more readily recognize key words, names, and so forth.
- If you know that a particular book, movie, or some other topic will be discussed, learn about it in

GINGER'S STORY: Coping beautifully

Virginia (Ginger) Zeller's journey with hearing trouble didn't begin with the usual struggle to hear words in conversation. Instead, it started during a hike in the 1990s, when Ginger began to hear crickets that weren't actually there. The problem was tinnitus, often referred to as "ringing in the ears." For her, however, it wasn't a ringing sound, but more like a cricket chirping.

The noise was so persistent and frustrating that she sought attention at Massachusetts Eye and Ear Infirmary, where she learned three things. First, her sensorineural hearing loss was mild enough that she didn't need hearing aids—at least, not yet. Second, her condition was progressive and would likely get much worse over time. And third, there really wasn't much she could do to make the cricket sounds go away, other than trying behavior modification techniques that, for her, didn't seem to do much good.

Since her mother had suffered from an acoustic neuroma, she went back for a hearing test every year. Five years after the trouble began, she was fitted for her first set of hearing aids. What she didn't expect was that not only did her hearing improve, but the cricket sounds also went away. That's actually a common occurrence for those with tinnitus. They experience relief with hearing aids, because the increased volume of the background noise helps to mask the sounds.

Now, at age 63, Ginger has been wearing hearing aids in both ears for about 12 years. As her hearing has gotten progressively worse, the hearing aids have gotten more powerful and more visible, but this is a nonissue for her. She welcomes each hearing aid change because she has found that if the hearing aid is not as powerful as it should be, the "crickets" come back.

The hearing aids, along with wireless technology that keeps her connected, have also brought the more common advantages one would expect, such as the ability to continue her career as an insurance broker. "I'm a people person, and without my hearing aids, I wouldn't be able to do my job," she says.

Unlike many who prefer their hearing aids to be hidden from view, Ginger wants people to notice her hearing aids, so that when they speak with her for the first time, they understand that she is hearing impaired without her having to explain it. She recalls one conversation where she was having difficulty understanding someone who was speaking. "Are you deaf?" the person asked in frustration. To that person's apparent shock, Ginger responded, "Yes, I am."

Ever resourceful, she's come up with several additional techniques that help her stay connected to her social world. She trained her Chihuahua, Pancho, to bark when she receives a text message or to let her know when someone is at the door. She also picks restaurants with low ceilings and good acoustics and arranges to be seated in a corner, where she can hear best.

As for people who don't want to wear hearing aids, she says, "They need to understand that if they don't wear their hearing aids, they are going to miss so much. I know that wearing them can be uncomfortable—and for most people it takes time to get used to the sound—but it's almost like getting your kids to eat broccoli. You may not like it at first, but eventually you will. I tell people, just wear them for a week and see what happens. It will be worth it."

advance. When you know what a person is talking about, it is easier to follow the conversation.
- When you are aware that you missed something that was said, ask that it be repeated.
- Use the highly rated Listening and Communication Enhancement (LACE) adaptive auditory training program (www.lacelistening.com). LACE is a software or Web-based program that helps individuals train their brains to hear better. The program helps people enhance their skills and strategies to deal with situations when hearing is inadequate.
- Consider joining your local chapter of the Hearing Loss Association of America (HLAA; see "Resources," page 48). HLAA provides information, advocacy, and support for people with hearing loss, including monthly group meetings that connect you to others with hearing loss.

If someone you know is hearing impaired

If you're not hearing impaired yourself, but are close to someone who is, there are several things that you can do to make communication as easy as possible.
- Speak in a normal tone of voice. Shouting distorts the sound of the voice.
- Talk slowly and clearly.
- Always face the person as you speak and position yourself three to six feet away so that he or she can read your lips for cues.
- If you think, based on the person's facial expressions, that he or she hasn't understood you, rephrase what you have just said.
- Ask the person if there is anything else you can do to make conversations easier. He or she may have suggestions that would help.

Preventing further hearing loss

It's never too late to start protecting your ears. Nothing will restore the hearing you had when you were 20, but you can make the most of the hearing that remains, and you can slow or halt further decline. The most important thing you can do is guard against loud noises. Any sound that's loud enough to hurt your ears, prompt temporary hearing loss, or cause ringing in the ears can destroy hair cells and lead to permanent hearing loss, whether it comes from leaf blowers, lawn mowers, wood chippers, chain saws, snow blowers, or noisy household appliances, like vacuum cleaners and blow dryers.

When you know you're going to be exposed to loud noise, wear earplugs, earmuffs, or both. Earplugs or earmuffs each can reduce the loudness of sounds by 15 to 30 dB. Earplugs work better against low-frequency noises, while earmuffs offer more protection against high-frequency noises. When you know you'll be exposed to noise louder than 105 dB for an extended period, wear earplugs and earmuffs together for the best protection. Examples of noise in this range include rock concerts, jet planes taking off or landing 100 feet away, and shotgun blasts (see Table 3, at left).

Another option is noise-canceling headphones, though these can be quite expensive. They work well for blocking low-frequency noises by creating a sound pattern opposite to the background noise, thus canceling it out.

If you use stereo headphones or earbuds, keep the volume at a reasonable level. Don't turn it up in an attempt to drown out other noise in the room. The volume on some portable stereos goes up to 126 dB, which is comparable to the ear-piercing noise of a jackhammer or chain saw. If you use earbuds, consider switching to headphones that muffle outside noise—that way, you can hear your music better at a moderate volume.

Aside from guarding against exposure to loud noise, you can take other steps to conserve your hearing. If you are hearing impaired, have your hearing checked yearly. If your hearing has deteriorated since your last test, it's important to know why, so that you can get proper treatment. For example, you may need to have your hearing aid reprogrammed or replaced with a new, more powerful one. Some experts think that maintaining a good level of hearing can slow further hearing loss by keeping the

Table 3: How loud is safe?
Protect your ears from sounds louder than 80 dB.

DECIBELS	SOUND
20	Watch ticking
30	Whispering
40	Leaves rustling, refrigerator humming
50	Neighborhood street, average home
60	Dishwasher, normal conversation
70	Car, alarm clock, city traffic
80	Garbage disposal, noisy restaurant, vacuum cleaner, outboard motor, hair dryer
85	Factory, screaming child, portable stereo at high volume
90	Power lawn mower, highway driving in a convertible
100	Diesel truck, subway train (outside, not as a passenger), chain saw
120	Rock concert, propeller plane, some portable stereos on maximum volume
130	Jet plane (100 feet away), air-raid siren
140	Shotgun blast, explosion

Sounds of 80 dB or less are believed to be safe for nearly all healthy adults, no matter how long you hear them. Sounds of 85 dB should be limited to no more than eight hours a day, and 91 dB to two hours for a healthy adult. Limit 100-dB sounds to 15 minutes and 120-dB sounds to about nine seconds. Sounds in the range of 125 to 140 dB are loud enough to cause pain unless you protect your ears with earplugs. The long-term health effects of high noise levels for children are unknown; therefore, the thresholds cited here may be too high for them.

brain attuned to signals from the auditory nerves.

Another way to prevent hearing loss is to be careful when cleaning your ears. The best way to clean your ears is to use a washcloth to wipe gently around the crevices. Soap and water work just fine. The ear irrigation systems sold over the counter in drugstores are also safe as long as you use them gently. Don't poke a washcloth or anything else into your ear deeper than the opening of the ear canal; otherwise, you may push earwax into the canal, where it can cause conductive hearing loss. Avoid using cotton swabs to clean your ears. Many people wind up in the doctor's office with injuries to the ear canals because they worked cotton swabs too far into their ears.

Finally, don't smoke. If you smoke, try to quit. Avoid being around others who are smoking. There's evidence that smoking and secondhand smoke can increase the risk of hearing loss, not to mention many other health problems as well. Research in animals has found nicotine-like receptors in hair cells, which suggests that smoking may be toxic to these cells. Smoking may also impair hearing by constricting blood vessels and restricting blood flow to the ears. Although some studies have not found a connection, most have noted that smokers are at an increased risk of hearing loss. ▼

Occupational hazards

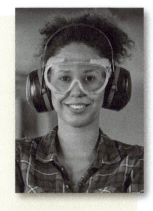

If you're exposed to loud noise on the job, you're entitled to certain protections from your employer. The Occupational Safety and Health Administration, which has the power under the federal government to regulate noise in the workplace, states that workers should not be exposed to constant noise above 90 dB for longer than eight hours. Companies with work areas that exceed this standard are required by law to have hearing-conservation programs that accomplish the following:

- Identify work areas with potentially hazardous noise levels.
- Take steps to control this noise.
- Schedule regular hearing screening tests of employees.
- Require employees to wear earplugs, earmuffs, or similar ear-protection devices.
- Educate workers on the dangers of loud noise.
- Make sure workers with hearing loss get the proper care to help prevent further hearing damage.

Using audio players safely

If you or someone you know wears earbuds frequently, be careful not to turn the volume up too high. Digital music players, with their long-lasting battery power and sound levels capable of reaching 115 dB, enable you to listen for hours upon hours to an endless stream of very loud music. Earbuds placed inside the ear canal boost sound delivered to the listener even more.

Researchers recommend limiting the amount of time spent listening to an hour a day at a volume level of around 6, if 10 is the highest volume. The more you turn down the volume, the longer you can listen. Noise-canceling headphones that block out background noise are helpful because you don't have to turn the volume as high to hear the music, but these are not always practical because they are expensive. Some people like to wirelessly connect their digital music players to speakers. Spending more time listening through speakers is better because the sound is diffused, and not delivered directly into the ear canal.

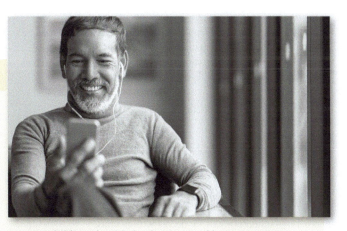

Younger children should also be aware of how to protect their hearing. The National Institute on Deafness and Other Communication Disorders maintains a website aimed at educating "tweens" ages 8 to 12 and their parents about noise-induced hearing loss.

For more information, visit the webpage of Noisy Planet public education campaign, a program developed by the National Institute on Deafness and Other Communication Disorders (part of the National Institutes of Health), at www.noisyplanet.nidcd.nih.gov.

Resources

Organizations

American Academy of Audiology
11480 Commerce Park Drive, Suite 220
Reston, VA 20190
800-222-2336 (toll-free)
www.audiology.org
www.HowsYourHearing.org (website for consumers)

The world's largest professional organization of audiologists, AAA provides information about audiograms and hearing aids. You can also get a list of audiologists in your area.

American Academy of Otolaryngology–Head and Neck Surgery
1650 Diagonal Road
Alexandria, VA 22314
703-836-4444
www.entnet.org

This medical society publishes patient education brochures on hearing loss. The website enables you to find a list of otolaryngologists in your area.

American Speech-Language-Hearing Association
2200 Research Blvd.
Rockville, MD 20850
Action Center: 800-638-8255 (toll-free)
TTY: 301-296-5700
www.asha.org

The national professional and accrediting organization of audiologists and speech and language pathologists, ASHA provides information about hearing disorders to consumers upon request. Using an online directory, you can find an audiologist or speech and language pathologist in your area.

American Tinnitus Association
P.O. Box 424049
Washington, DC 20042
800-634-8978 (toll-free)
www.ata.org

This nonprofit organization supports scientific research on tinnitus, provides consumer information about the condition, and organizes support groups for people with tinnitus.

Hearing Education and Awareness for Rockers
P.O. Box 460847
San Francisco, CA 94146
415-409-3277
24-hour hotline: 415-773-9590
www.hearnet.com

A nonprofit organization, HEAR is dedicated to raising awareness of the dangers of repeated exposure to excessive noise levels for musicians, fans, or anyone concerned about hearing problems.

Hearing Loss Association of America
7910 Woodmont Ave., Suite 1200
Bethesda, MD 20814
301-657-2248
www.hearingloss.org

This patient-advocacy group provides information on hearing loss, hearing aids, and medical treatments. It also maintains local support groups and works with federal, state, and local governments on laws to benefit hearing-impaired people.

International Hearing Society
16880 Middlebelt Road, Suite 4
Livonia, MI 48154
734-522-7200
www.ihsinfo.org

This is the professional and certifying organization for hearing aid dispensers. IHS provides a list of board-certified hearing instrument specialists in your area. You can email a question from the website.

National Institute on Deafness and Other Communication Disorders
31 Center Drive, MSC 2320
Bethesda, MD 20892
800-241-1044 (toll-free)
TTY: 800-241-1055 (toll-free)
www.nidcd.nih.gov

This branch of the National Institutes of Health provides information on research and ways to protect against hearing loss.

Books

The Consumer Handbook on Hearing Loss and Noise
Marshall Chasin, Au.D., editor
(Auricle Ink Publishers, 2010)

In this book, doctors and other experts address different aspects of noise-induced hearing loss, including the basics of noise and hearing, ways to improve communication in the presence of noise, architectural strategies to minimize noise, legal issues surrounding noise-induced hearing loss, and other health problems caused by noise.

Shouting Won't Help: Why I—and 50 Million Other Americans—Can't Hear You
Katherine Bouton
(Sarah Crichton Books, 2013)

A former editor at *The New York Times* chronicles her experiences with sensorineural hearing loss, after she suddenly went deaf in her left ear. In addition to detailing her own story (which includes hearing aids and a cochlear implant), she seeks out doctors, audiologists, neurobiologists, and other people who've suffered from hearing loss, to illuminate different aspects of the problem.